Medical Futility

A Cross-National Study

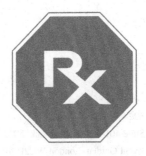

Medical Futility

A Cross-National Study

edited by

Alireza Bagheri, MD, PhD
Tehran University of Medical Sciences, Iran

foreword by

Daniel Callahan, PhD
The Hastings Center, USA

Imperial College Press

ICP

Published by

Imperial College Press
57 Shelton Street
Covent Garden
London WC2H 9HE

Distributed by

World Scientific Publishing Co. Pte. Ltd.
5 Toh Tuck Link, Singapore 596224
USA office: 27 Warren Street, Suite 401-402, Hackensack, NJ 07601
UK office: 57 Shelton Street, Covent Garden, London WC2H 9HE

Library of Congress Cataloging-in-Publication Data
Bagheri, Alireza.
    Medical futility : a cross-national study / by Alireza Bagheri.
       p. ; cm.
    Includes bibliographical references and index.
    ISBN 978-1-84816-990-6 (hardcover : alk. paper)
    I. Title.
    [DNLM: 1. Life Support Care--ethics. 2. Medical Futility. 3. Cross-Cultural Comparison.
4. Health Policy. 5. Terminal Care--ethics. 6. Terminal Care--legislation & jurisprudence. WB 60]

    174.2'96029--dc23

                                                        2012046672

British Library Cataloguing-in-Publication Data
A catalogue record for this book is available from the British Library.

Typeset by Stallion Press
Email: enquiries@stallionpress.com

Printed in Singapore

For Maryam, Sareh and Ava

CONTENTS

ABOUT THE EDITOR

Alireza Bagheri-chimeh, MD, PhD, is assistant professor of medicine and medical ethics, School of Medicine, Tehran University of Medical Sciences, Iran. Since 2005, Dr. Bagheri has been conducting empirical studies on medical futility in several countries such as Japan, Korea, Canada, the United States and Iran. He is a Physician from Iran (1993) with a PhD degree in medical ethics from Japan (2004). His work on end-of-life issues, concentrating on brain death and organ transplantation, began in 1998. His research into medical futility started when he was a fellow at the School of Law, Kyoto University in 2005, and then in 2007, under the tutelage of Professor Edmund Pellegrino, a fellow of Georgetown University, USA. Dr. Bagheri broadened his scope on end-of-life clinical ethics consultation during his clinical ethics fellowship at the Joint Center for Bioethics, University of Toronto, Canada.

In 2010, Dr. Bagheri received the National Razi (Rhazes) Medical Research Award for his work on medical futility. His experience in working as a palliative care doctor in Iran and then gaining experience in this area in Canada helped him to understand the complexity of the issue not only as a clinical ethicist but also as a physician with experience in handling difficulties relating to futility decision making. Dr. Bagheri is currently the Vice-Chairman of the UNESCO International Bioethics Committee (IBC) and a member of the board of directors of the International Association of Bioethics (IAB).

CONTRIBUTORS

Said Abuhasna is Clinical Professor in Medical Health Sciences at the United Arab Emirates University, and Chief of ICU, Chairman of the Department of Critical Care Medicine and Chairman of the Ethics Committee at Tawam Hospital. He is a member of the Editorial Board of *World Journal of Trauma and Critical Care Medicine* and the journal *Anaesthesia, Pain and Intensive Care* (APIC).

Ahmet Acıduman is Associate Professor of Medicine and History of Medicine and Ethics, Faculty of Medicine, Ankara University, Turkey. He is a member of the Turkish Neurosurgical Society, Turkish Bioethics Association, Society of Medical Ethics and Medical Law and International Association for Education in Ethics.

Ali Abdulkareem Al Obaidli is an internist and nephrologist trained at the University of Toronto and completed his MPH at the Johns Hopkins Bloomberg School of Public Health. He is currently working as a nephrologist at Sheikh Khalifa Medical City and is Chief Clinical Officer for Abu Dhabi Health Services (SEHA), United Arab Emirates.

Atsushi Asai is Professor of Medicine and Bioethics at the Department of Bioethics, Kumamoto University Graduate School of Medicine, Kumamoto, Japan. He was visiting research fellow, Centre for Human Bioethics, Monash University in Australia and also ethics fellow in the University of California, in San Francisco, USA.

Lieven Annemans is Professor of Health Economics at the medical faculties of Ghent University and Brussels University. He is former President of the International Society for Pharmacoeconomics and Outcomes Research, and a current member of the Flemish Strategic Council for Health and Wellbeing.

Berna Arda is Professor of Medical Ethics and History of Medicine, School of Medicine, Ankara University, Turkey. She was a founding chairperson of the Turkish Bioethics Society (1994–2001), and is a member of the High Disciplinary Committee of the Turkish Medical Association. She is Governor and Vice-president of the World Association for Medical Law, and Chair of the Board of Directors of the International Association for Education in Ethics.

Alireza Bagheri is Assistant Professor of Medicine and Medical Ethics, School of Medicine, Tehran University of Medical Sciences, Iran. He is Vice-chairman of the UNESCO International Bioethics Committee (IBC) and a member of the board of directors of the International Association of Bioethics (IAB).

Jan L Bernheim is a medical oncologist and Emeritus Professor of Medicine at the Vrije Universiteit Brussel (VUB). In 1979 he co-founded the first palliative care unit in Belgium and the Quality of Life Study Group of the European Organization for Research and Treatment of Cancer. He is a senior member of the End-of-Life Care Research Group of the VUB and University of Ghent and of the Coma Science Group of the University of Liège.

Daniel Callahan is President Emeritus of The Hastings Center and was its co-founder in 1969. He is the author most recently of *In Search of the Good: A Life in Bioethics* and *The Roots of Bioethics: Health, Progress, Technology, Death*. He received his PhD in philosophy from Harvard.

Gabriel d'Empaire is Professor of Bioethics in Central University of Venezuela and Director of Coronary and Intensive Care Unit, Clínicas Caracas Hospital. Dr. d'Empaire is the President of the Bioethics Clinical Association of Venezuela and a guest member of the National Academy of Medicine of Venezuela. He was a member of the UNESCO International Bioethics Committee (2004–2011).

Qingli Hu is Professor of Medicine and a member of the Bioethics Expert Committee, Ministry of Health, China. He is Emeritus Professor at Shanghai Jiaotong University School of Medicine. He is a member of the UNESCO International Bioethics Committee.

Yasuhiro Kadooka is a medical doctor and research fellow in the Department of Bioethics, Kumamoto University Graduate School of

Medicine, Kumamoto, Japan. During his PhD course on bioethics he has explored the issue of medical futility in Japan.

Tanja Krones is Physician of the University of Zurich, Institute of Biomedical Ethics, University Hospital of Zurich, Clinical Ethics, Switzerland.

Olga I Kubar is Professor of Medicine and Head of the Clinical Department at the Institut Pasteur in Saint Petersburg, Russia. She is a member of the UNESCO International Bioethics Committee (IBC).

Ivo Kwon is Director of the Ewha Center for Medical Ethics and Humanities, School of Medicine, Ewha Womans University, and Professor in the Department of Medical Education, School of Medicine, Ewha Womans University, Korea.

Cunfang Mao is President of the Shanghai Health Professionals Association, China; and Vice President of the *Shanghai Medical and Pharmaceutical Journal*, China.

Dominique Martin is a Bioethicist at the Centre for Health and Society in the University of Melbourne, where she currently lectures in Health Ethics. She has previously worked as a medical practitioner in Emergency Medicine. Her research interests include issues concerning the procurement and use of human biological materials and issues in professional ethics for healthcare practitioners.

Galina L Mikirtichian is Professor of Medicine and Head of the Medical Humanities and Bioethics Department, St. Petersburg State Pediatric Medical Academy, Russia.

Settimio Monteverde is a PhD candidate at the Institute of Biomedical Ethics at the University of Zurich (Careum Fellow) and Lecturer for Nursing Ethics in the Division of Health, Bern University of Applied Sciences, Switzerland.

Marina I Petrova is Medical Director of the St. Olga Hospice at the St. Petersburg City Hospital, Russia.

Leo Pessini is Professor of Bioethics at Saint Camillus University Center, Sao Paulo, Brazil. He is Editor of *Ibero-American Bioethics, History and Perspectives* (2010) and Co-editor of the journal *Bioethikos*. He is currently President of the Camillian Organization in Brazil.

William Saad Hossne is Emeritus Professor at the State University Sao Paulo in Botucatu and ex-President of the National Commission for Ethics of Research Involving Human Subjects in Brazil. He is Coordinator of the Post-graduate Program in Bioethics at Saint Camillus University Center and Co-editor of the journal *Bioethikos*.

Yongxing Shi is Executive Deputy Director of Life Care Research Center, China Association for Life Care. He is also Director of the Care for Elderly Society Shanghai Health Professionals Association and Dean of the Hospice of Zhabei District, Shanghai, China.

Thierry Vansweevelt is Professor of Tort Law and Medical Law at the University of Antwerp, Belgium. He is Editor of the bilingual Belgian *Journal of Health Law*. He is also a lawyer at the law firm Dewallens & Partners.

Robert M Veatch is Professor of Medical Ethics and former Director of the Kennedy Institute of Ethics, Georgetown University. He was an expert witness for the mother in the case of Baby K and has criticized physicians who make normative futility decisions while accepting their role in deciding physiological futility.

Yang Yang is Lecturer, Dalian Medical University, China; Editor, *Journal of Medicine and Philosophy*, China; and Secretary, Youth Committee of Philosophy of Medicine Association.

Mingjie Zhao is President of the Press of Dalian Medical University, Routine Editor-in-Chief of the *Journal of Medicine and Philosophy*, China, and Professor, Doctoral Advisor on Medical Humanities, Dalian Medical University.

Hui Zhu is Assistant Director of Life Care Research Center, Shanghai, China.

ACKNOWLEDGMENTS

I would like to thank my colleagues for their scholarly contributions to this book. They have successfully provided an international scope on medical futility. My thanks also to the anonymous reviewers whose comments helped to improve the quality of the discussion in each chapter.

In this regard, I would like to thank Alastair Campbell and Alexander Capron, for their valuable reviews and comments. My special thanks to Dan Callahan, one of the pioneers of this topic, for his invaluable foreword to this book.

The idea for this book came about when I was the Edmund Pellegrino Fellow at the Center for Clinical Bioethics in Georgetown University, Washington DC. I am forever indebted to Dr. Pellegrino who provided me with continuous encouragement and guidance.

FOREWORD

IS THE FUTILITY DEBATE FUTILE?

When I published an article in 1991 on the problem of futility, the concept had by then (at least in the United States) been taken up by many as a way out of difficult ethical dilemmas of end-of-life care. The idea that physician efforts to extend life could be ended when there was no further benefit to patients had a long history prior to that time. But "benefit" was a term that could be interpreted in different ways and was often a source of disagreement. The seemingly apparent advantage of the word "futile" was that it had about it a kind of scientific flavor, something that could be dealt with as a standard medical problem, not requiring ethical analysis. The dictionary defines "futile" as "useless" or "ineffectual," and the word could easily be used, so it was thought, to make yes or no, black or white decisions. Many people die every day and there is just nothing that medicine can do about that in many cases. Futility as a standard would make end-of-life care decisions easier, and who could not welcome that possibility? But it wasn't that simple, as the ensuing discussion and debate unfolded. Did futile mean zero probability of benefit, as many felt, or a very low probability of benefit, but not zero probability? At the extreme it could be pointed out that there are no beneficial treatments for decapitation, that it meets the zero probability standard. But what about situations where the probability of benefit is 0.005%, exceedingly low, and, we could well say, quite improbable — but not impossible. And thus, by the standard dictionary definition, not useless. What then should we do with probabilities?

Those further debates began to make clear that a decision about futility is not one that can be reduced to some simple scientific, medical judgment. Technological developments have made it increasingly difficult to say that there is, except for comparatively rare situations, some decisively sharp line between futile and non-futile. It is more accurate to say that the care of the dying almost always requires a grappling with probabilities, that is, with a range of possibilities that are a function of available technologies that can extend life, even if only for minutes or hours; different patient physical resiliency characteristics; and (sometimes) the medical skills of doctors in dealing with critical illness. Every physician can tell a story about some patient whose treatment at some point seemed futile by ordinary medical practice standards, but it was continued against all odds — and the patient survived.

I have come, that is, to think that the concept of futility cannot work the kind of diagnostic magic many thought it could two decades ago. Yet despite the difficulties it raises I believe it has been a concept worthy of analysis and use. The question of what counts as a benefit of treatment is both old and ever new, and futility is one way to think about it in end-of-life care. The essays collected in this valuable volume, *Medical Futility: A Cross-National Study*, show that there is no common universal standard for the concept of futility or its proper use. But the debate about its meaning, and its various uses in different cultures and countries, has been valuable.

End-of-life care has, I believe, become harder not easier in recent years because of medicine's power to keep sick and dying patients alive for longer times, often too much longer. Some treatments are indeed useless. It is just that it is harder to say just when that happens and just which they are. These essays give us some useful, interesting, and insightful ways to cope with that problem, which I suspect will not end in the near, or maybe even in the far, future.

Daniel Callahan
President Emeritus of
The Hastings Center, USA

INTRODUCTION

The concept of medical futility has been a part of medicine since its inception, as medical science has always been limited in its ability to cure diseases. Therefore, medical futility is in fact an acknowledgement that there is a point in a patient's treatment when medicine is powerless. A point at which patients are overcome by their diseases; the point which tells us "enough is enough."

For healthcare professionals, it can be a difficult ethical dilemma to determine when to withdraw or withhold treatments deemed futile. Conflicts may arise when physicians and patients have differing ideas about the goals of treatment. There can also be tension when care providers receive requests for futile therapies from patients or their families. In a multicultural setting, cultural differences may lead to misunderstandings about the goals of treatment, which can make decision making particularly complex. It can be difficult to negotiate transitions from aggressive treatment to comfort care with patients and their families.

Medical futility, once called "a problem without a name" (Callahan 1991), is a controversial issue in its definition and in its applications. The controversy exists, partly, in disagreements between families and physicians about goals of treatment and the ends of medicine.

The ends of medicine, if defined clearly, would determine when medical intervention is meaningful and when further treatment is beyond the powers of medicine. This would guide healthcare professionals on how vigorously to treat and about when it is morally permissible to withhold or withdraw life-sustaining treatment. However, the controversy about the ends of medicine

1

gives different answers to this question, and therefore the controversy about medical futility, in its definition and application, refers partly to the controversy over the end of medicine. The inevitability of human death, limitations of medical science, scarcity of health resources, and various socio-cultural issues mean that decisions regarding end-of-life care in general, and medical futility in particular, are an inescapable reality in clinical settings throughout the world. As Dr. Pellegrino reminds, "there is a time when medical interventions are no longer serving the good of the patient, when the good is no longer attainable, the intervention in question is futile; i.e., it cannot attain the desired goal. This is when physician, patient, and/or family must confront the universal fact of human finitude" (Pellegrino 2005).

It should be noted that the relevance of medical futility might differ from country to country. In industrial countries, medical futility is an important issue because of their relatively aged populations. However, in developing countries, it is an important issue because of the scarcity of health resources. It also should be stressed that medical futility is not limited to the end-of-life context. Physicians frequently conduct examinations, or prescribe treatments or drugs to reassure the patient or to satisfy a patient's request, without any medical indication (Baily 2011). Although discussions about medical futility began almost three decades ago in the United States, there are few books dedicated to this important issue, and existing books have mostly focused on the American context. Literature about medical futility from other countries is scarce. More information is required to determine the impact of the problem in different healthcare systems, and to learn more about how this problem is addressed around the world. This book elucidates the concept of medical futility and demonstrates the application of futility to practical patient care decisions in different healthcare systems.

Authors from 13 different developed and developing countries have contributed to this volume, examining how fee-for-service, capitation payment models, and insurance plans affect approaches to medical futility. It also explains how socio-cultural and moral views are superimposed on financial considerations. Several contributions show how developing regulations or guidelines may help physicians make decisions about futile treatments, potentially decreasing disagreements between healthcare providers and patients' family members. Such guidelines can help healthcare professionals decide how aggressively to treat patients. They may also help physicians make decisions about when it is morally permissible to withhold or withdraw futile treatments.

Existing controversy about the proper goals of medicine has been cited as an obstacle to regulating medical futility. However, medical futility cannot be defined independently from medical facts, normative values, and socio-economic considerations. Any attempt to develop an operational definition or guidelines must include the opinions of patients and families. Such policies should be based on neither excessive patient autonomy nor physician paternalism (Bagheri 2008). This approach may lead to ethically and morally viable solutions. A sound policy should emphasize the establishment of a constructive and informative dialogue to help each party to come to understand the other's concerns. This approach encourages all parties to understand and accept the limits of medicine and the inescapable clinical reality in which they should no longer rely on their personal views alone. Physicians should listen to their patient's concerns and the patient/family should realize the limits of medicine and respect the just claims of others on scarce resources.

Each chapter has been structured to describe medical futility in the contributors' countries by providing information about five issues: (1) the country's healthcare system, including its payment system (e.g. capitation or fee-for-service/insurance policy) and how the payment system may affect decision making about medical futility; (2) ethics in end-of-life issues in their society; (3) legislation and guidelines, professional codes and protocols that address medical futility; (4) the nature of decision making regarding futile care; and (5) how medical futility is distinguished or linked to euthanasia in their country. This structure enables easy comparisons between countries.

In a scholarly article from the United States, Robert Veatch reminds us that the central moral issue of futile treatment is whether, independent of resource issues, there are moral arguments unique to this class of treatments that justify a physician's refusal to provide or, alternatively, support a patient's right of access to futile treatment.

The article provides deep insight into medical futility, including its definition and different classifications — physiological and normative — as well as the history of the futility debate in the United States. He explains how two US states (Texas and Virginia) have attempted to address the issue through legislative and regulatory approaches and allow a physician to unilaterally withhold or withdraw life-sustaining treatments against the wishes of the patient or surrogate. Veatch reveals that almost all court cases regarding futile treatment advocate patients' and surrogates' rights to access futile treatments, provided specified conditions are met.

An analytical article from Brazil shows how legal concern may compel physicians to have a more aggressive attitude to provide futile treatment at the end of life, despite their belief that this approach may not be the best for the patient. The authors describe the challenges of harmonizing judicial rulings with ethical standards in a country with laws and regulations to manage end-of-life issues.

Belgium is unique in having both legalized physician-assisted dying and the most developed palliative care program in Europe. Bernheim and his colleagues describe how these factors reduce instances of medically futile treatments at the end of life. The article explains that euthanasia has been widely integrated into comprehensive palliative care, thus reducing demand for futile treatments. It shows how statistical data from epidemiological studies can be used in the development of end-of-life care policies.

The contribution from Venezuela describes how physicians define futile treatments as those which do not benefit patients, while exploring challenges related to cultural and linguistic differences. The author explains that the lack of unified medical protocol causes great variation in the way that physicians approach medical futility.

In Chapter 5 a review of the issue in the Russian Federation shows how the term "futile medicine" is absent from the vocabulary of medical professionals, and therefore all ethical, social, legal and medical aspects associated with end-of-life treatment and medical futility are expressed through the concept of palliative medicine. The article describes decisions about futile treatment framed within the context of palliative care. In this approach, physicians should act in the patient's best interests while setting therapeutic goals for the patient. That means physicians treat their patients within reasonable limits of available health resources while acknowledging the natural processes of human death. The authors argue that there are no objective criteria to withdraw end-of-life treatment, noting the importance of determining the appropriate time to transition to comprehensive palliative care if aggressive interventions are futile.

The article from Australia provides not only the author's perspective on medical futility, but it also provides a review of the issue in her country. The article discusses the role of palliative care and describes how decisions about medical futility are a key issue in the Australian healthcare system.

In Chapter 7, the authors explain that medical futility is an immediate problem in Japan that must be addressed by the Japanese healthcare system. They examine aspects of the Japanese healthcare system that have led to lengthy hospitalizations, frequent medical examinations, and overtreatment of the elderly. The article describes factors that have caused a rise in demand on Japan's healthcare system, including an aging population, advances in medical technology, and cost-containment measures, including the introduction of a flat-fee payment system causing a rise in national health expenditure. The article explains why Japanese physicians are hesitant to forgo life-prolonging treatments for terminally ill patients. In clinical settings, most end-of-life decisions have been left to individual doctors because there is no institutional system to deal with controversial issues in a team context. It demonstrates how Japanese views on life and death are influenced by the Shinto religion. Interestingly, a public survey by the Japanese Ministry of Health confirmed that most of the population is not in favor of aggressive life-prolonging treatments deemed futile. The authors explain how in deciding to withdraw life-prolonging treatments for terminally ill patients, many Japanese physicians confront legal, emotional, and cultural barriers.

In the article from China, Yongxing Shi and colleagues describe how the great challenge in terminal care is the traditional Chinese view of death, which holds that the end of life is inauspicious and the greatest "evil". In Chinese society, the idea of "cherishing life but dreading death" has influenced the attitudes of the public and physicians in decision making about medical futility.

Authors explain the moral dilemma between the traditional medical ethics of "retrieving the dying and rescuing the wounded" and requests to prolong patients' lives by applying modern medical technology despite beliefs that such treatment is futile. This also explains how overtreatment is relatively common in China.

The contribution from Korea explains how withdrawing futile treatment from dying patients is understood as "death with dignity", which means facing death in harmony with the natural order. The article shows how in end-of-life decision making, the patient's wishes may sometimes be overridden by the wishes of family members. It also confirms that end-of-life decisions are sometimes influenced by the economic burden faced by families due to the insufficiency of the national health insurance system.

Chapter 10 provides insight into medical futility in Switzerland by comparing it with the situations in Germany and the United States. The authors explain how in the "Swiss approach", futility decisions are based on societal and economic elements with a strong reliance on risk-benefit assessments by individual physicians. The article elaborates how, since the enactment of the Health Insurance Law, different cases involving the refusal of insurers or the state to pay for interventions deemed medically futile have drawn public attention. It explains how in one case, the Federal Supreme Court ruled that the insurer was not obliged to cover the costs of the futile treatment because it did not offer a substantial therapeutic benefit, and cost-effectiveness could not be demonstrated.

In Chapter 11, the authors indicate that in Turkey, death-related discussions are extremely limited, and the subject is discussed very little during medical school and specialty training. The article explains that in Turkey — as is the case in many countries — there is a lack of studies examining how physicians make end-of-life decisions, and whether or not social factors affect these decisions. According to the Patients' Rights Act of 1998, physicians have the right not to offer medically futile interventions if the patient does not "need" the treatment. This right is also based on considerations of fair resource allocation.

The articles from Iran and the United Arab Emirates (UAE) show how religious beliefs and Islamic teachings are important in end-of-life decision making, especially in cases of futile treatment. An empirical survey in Iran shows that scarcity of medical resources, the patient's suffering, the family's opinion and religious concerns are four influential factors in futility decisions. It shows how physicians and health policy makers are focusing attention on the need to develop guidelines regarding medical futility.

In the UAE, a lack of understanding about the prognosis of terminal illnesses leads patients' families to request futile treatments. The authors explain how the idea of limiting futile treatment is gaining acceptance among families and physicians.

This book is intended to deepen our understanding of medical futility by examining the approaches and experiences of nations with different cultures, healthcare systems, and socio-economic statuses. It offers valuable insights for countries where medical futility is becoming a critical issue. It calls on us to distinguish between futile treatments, which do not benefit patients, with concerns about allocating resources in ways that can produce more good if they are used for other patients. A deeper understanding of these issues, along with sound guidelines, can help physicians approach cases of medical futility in a way that is morally sound.

Alireza Bagheri
Toronto, November 3, 2012

REFERENCES

Bagheri A. 2008. Regulating medical futility: Neither physician's paternalism, nor excessive patient's autonomy. *European Journal of Health Law* 15: 45–53.

Baily MA. 2011. Futility, autonomy, and cost in end-of-life care. *Journal of Law, Medicine And Ethics* 39: 172–182.

Callahan D. 1991. Medical futility, medical necessity: The-problem-without-a-name. *Hastings Center Report* 21: 30–35.

Pellegrino E. 2005. Futility in medicine decisions: The word and the concept. *HEC FORUM* 17: 308–318.

CHAPTER ONE

SO-CALLED FUTILE CARE: THE EXPERIENCE OF THE UNITED STATES

Robert M Veatch

SUMMARY

By the mid-twentieth century most people in the United States were committed to preserving life whenever possible, but that soon was questioned. Even physicians, among the most dedicated to aggressive treatment, began to question such practices. When patients occasionally insisted on such efforts, physicians began demanding the right to unilaterally forgo life support, treatment they called "futile." The debate that followed and the cases and legal activities are presented here along with the critical conceptual distinctions. Physiological futility must be distinguished from normative futility and both kinds of cases separated from resource allocation concerns. The two most important cases — Helga Wanglie and Baby K — are presented as well as the one case in which the American courts have sided with the physician. The odd futility law of the state of Texas, which authorizes limited unilateral physician decisions to forgo life support, will be summarized as well. The limited role of the physician and more complex role of the family are presented and medical futility is compared to the broader issue of euthanasia in the United States.

INTRODUCTION

There was a time, about a half century ago, that Americans (and most people around the world) believed that human life should always be preserved, even when such efforts were burdensome and likely to fail. The last decades of the twentieth century saw radical change in that commitment. With the development of technologies that could stabilize what had previously been inevitably acutely fatal illness, Americans began rethinking their personal preferences and moral views. Views changed so rapidly that within about 20 years most people in the United States began to question the wisdom of preserving life in the face of terminal or serious chronic illness. Even physicians, who had been among the most militantly committed to preserving life, joined the "death with dignity" movement and conceded the appropriateness of making explicit and conscious decisions to forgo life-sustaining medical treatments. This shift was affirmed in the 1983 US government Commission report *Deciding to Forego Life Support* (President's Commission for the Study of Ethical Problems in Medicine and Biomedical and Behavioral Research 1983).

At the same time, the United States is extremely pluralistic. Even though a substantial consensus of health professionals and lay people began to affirm decisions to forgo, several minorities dissented, remaining militantly committed to preserving life even in cases in which efforts were inevitably going to fail. Orthodox Jews, some members of pro-life groups, and some minority ethnic groups tended to resist the emerging consensus. This would eventually lead to clashes between those who held these minority views and mainstream health professionals, at least mainstream professionals who had bought into the cultural acceptance of death while retaining the more traditional view that physicians should remain the authoritative decision-makers regarding medical decisions. By the last decade of the twentieth century several of these clashes were between patients or their surrogates who wanted maximal efforts to preserve life and physicians who thought it was wise to stop such efforts.

These clashes are often referred to as the futile care debate (Council on Ethical and Judicial Affairs, American Medical Association 1999; Jecker and Schneiderman 1993; Lantos *et al.* 1988; Lantos *et al.* 1989; Rubin 1998; Schneiderman, Jecker, and Jonsen 1990; Veatch and Spicer 1992; Youngner 1990; Youngner 1988).

THE HEALTHCARE SYSTEM IN THE UNITED STATES

The emergence of the futile care debate in the United States is, in part, to be attributed to its unique health care system. American culture prides itself on a "non-socialized," free-enterprise, individualistic health care that rejects a governmental health service or insurance. Individuals are, in theory, supposed to be responsible for their own health care and free to choose any insurance or fee-for-service delivery system. The bulk of the American population is covered by private health insurance provided by the employer of the head of each household.

At the same time, a large portion of the American public, in fact, gets government-funded or government-managed health insurance. Government accounts for 17 percent of the nation's workforce (Newman 2012), almost all of whom receive health insurance through government programs. The military, for example, receive health care through the Civilian Health and Medical Program of the Uniformed Services (CHAMPUS) (recently renamed TRICARE). It covers military personnel, retirees, and dependents. Virtually all persons over age 65 as well as those with disabilities are insured by the federal government Medicare system. It covers some 47 million people of a population numbering 313 million for either hospital or hospital plus medical services. In addition, Medicaid, a federally funded program administered by the states, covers 53 million low-income people. Some 50 million people are uninsured. A small number with means may self-pay, but many of these receive some level of charity care from hospitals and health professionals. Those covered by private insurance have their insurance heavily regulated by government agencies. Thus, the myth of a private free market in health care services is seriously misleading.

Moreover, each of these forms of medical service delivery may reflect a variety of payment systems, including fee-for-service, capitation, and health maintenance organizations, often including the commitment to provide "medically necessary" services for a fixed yearly fee (often with some combination of co-payments, deductibles, or expenditure caps). Medicare compensates hospitals with a fixed fee based on diagnosis and treatment combinations regardless of the actual costs to the hospital for any particular patient.

This complex, multi-dimensional health care system generates equally complex incentives related to so-called futile care. Private, fee-for-service practitioners and hospitals, in theory, have financial incentives to over-treat, in part by encouraging or at least going along with patient and family requests for life-sustaining services that doctors would recognize as futile. On the other hand, private insurance and health maintenance organizations (as well as government health care system managers) have incentives to minimize costs by refusing to fund services deemed futile.

Superimposed on these financial incentives is a set of cultural, moral views that affect delivery of medical care some would classify as futile. Conservative religious and cultural groups identifying with "pro-life" views may insist that all human life is precious and to be preserved even if the extension of life is transient and costly. In the past two decades doctors' groups have begun to insist that delivery of medical services deemed futile conflicts with the fundamental end of the practice of medicine. Proponents of this view insist the goal of medicine is to heal and that services that merely temporarily prolong the dying process are not part of the essence of good medicine. These governmental, financial, and cultural forces have clashed over the norms for delivery of medical services that are believed merely to prolong temporarily the life of the dying patient.

THE ETHICS OF END-OF-LIFE ISSUES
IN THE UNITED STATES

The ethical debates over futile care emerged in the late 1980s and early 1990s superimposed on an earlier and broader robust debate over end-of-life issues in the United States. Beginning in about 1970 patients began demanding a greater say in decisions about end-of-life care. In particular, they demanded the right to refuse medical treatments that they thought were merely prolonging the dying process without offering net benefits for the patient. These demands were often couched in terms of the right of the patient to refuse consent to medical treatment, a right embedded in the larger informed consent discussion. Many would see this movement as an outgrowth of the American and world-wide emergence of rights movements of the 1960s and 1970s (Veatch 2009). This period produced in the United States a civil rights movement, an anti-war movement, a women's rights movement, a student movement. Could a patients' rights movement be far behind?

Reliance on concepts of liberal political philosophy and law quickly led to replacing the more traditional, paternalistic physician-dominated decision-making (often committed to preserving life) with a more rights-oriented, patient-centered perspective recognizing the right of the patient to refuse any medical treatment whatsoever provided that treatment was offered for the patient's own good. (Hence, forced medical treatments for public health purposes were still considered acceptable, in principle.) Naturally, the treatments refused were often end-of-life interventions deemed of no net value by the patient.

This patients' rights perspective quickly prevailed as long as physicians were insisting on providing life support to patients who were refusing it. The perspective was more complicated, however, as physicians began to concur with the judgment that certain end-of-life interventions did more harm than good. In particular, in cases in which patients with minority views demanded life-prolonging care while physicians adopted the dominant interpretation that these interventions were pointless, the patients' rights perspective caused some confusion. Some apparently thought that, because a patients' rights perspective gave patients the right to refuse treatment, they also had a right to gain access even against the wishes of the physician. These cases began emerging in hospital settings in the late 1980s and soon led to court cases litigating the question of whether patients had a right of access to such treatments and whether physicians were required to deliver them.

Physiological vs. Normative Futility

The initial presumption that patients' rights required not only honoring a patient's right to refuse treatment, but also honoring his or her right of access was quickly challenged. Some physicians claimed, inappropriately, that deciding whether a treatment was useful or futile was entirely a matter of medical expertise. It was the doctor's call. Just as physicians had expertise that led them to have the authority to prescribe medications based on their knowledge of the pharmacology, toxicity, and treatment effects of drugs, so they had the authority to decide whether a treatment was useful or futile for the patient's condition.

This claim quickly generated much confusion and led to important conceptual clarifications. Many of us working in medical ethics had been insisting for decades that physicians could not legitimately claim expertise in deciding whether a particular treatment effect was a good or bad effect (Veatch 1973). Starting with a simple version of the classic fact/value dichotomy, we claimed that physicians could rightly claim expertise on the effects of a treatment, but could not go on to claim that the effect was good or bad. These judgments, we argued, were matters of evaluation requiring judgments that any human being was capable of making. Hence, the question of whether adding a week of unconscious life to a patient served a useful purpose was something any person — lay or professional — was capable of evaluating and rendering a judgment upon. This evaluative judgment had to be separated from the more technical, scientific question of whether an intervention would, in fact, extend life for a week, and, if so, at what probability.

Physiological Futility

This basic fact/value distinction led to a critical conceptual distinction in the futile care debate. We distinguished two kinds of futility: physiological and normative (Youngner 1988). The distinction rests on the nature of the disagreement between physician and patient. In some cases, the two parties are in agreement over the goal of the treatment and disagree over whether there is evidence that the treatment under consideration will achieve that goal or the probability it will be achieved. For example, patient and physician may agree that the goal is to eliminate an infection in the inner ear that is with a high degree of certainty viral. They are discussing whether an antibiotic will eliminate the infection. We would say they agree on the goal, but are disputing the facts of whether an antibiotic will achieve that goal. The claim of the physician would be that antibiotics will not have a physiological effect on the viral infection. The dispute is over the medical facts; not over the goal.

In such cases, there is widespread agreement that the physician legitimately claims expertise on matters of physiological futility. Of course, a physician may be in error (claiming, for example, that antibiotics eliminate the virus under consideration when there is no such evidence). The general claim, however, is that the physician is the presumed expert on such claims of medical fact. He or she is subject to the normal standards of peer review and could be accused of malpractice if an error is made on such factual matters. Generally, the patient is not authoritative in such disputes.

Moreover, in disputes over physiological futility the working presumption is that no physician has any obligation to deliver a treatment simply because the patient believes it will effectively produce the result the patient is seeking even if the expert opinion of the physician is to the contrary. Professionals could not function if they were obliged to deliver every treatment a patient demanded even if the overwhelming evidence was that it could not produce the effect the patient was seeking.

Normative Futility

By contrast, other disputes over futility are over the value of a goal that might be pursued. Consider the case of a patient diagnosed as permanently vegetative in which the patient (through an advanced directive) or a familial surrogate insists the life is still precious and should be preserved by medical intervention. A physician who disagrees and calls the intervention "futile" is not disagreeing over the factual matter of whether some life support will, in fact, extend life. There may well be agreement that the unconscious life could be extended, at least for a short period. The parties are not disputing the facts; they disagree about the value of the extension of life.

This second kind of disagreement is typically referred to as a dispute over normative futility. The parties agree on the facts, but dispute the value judgment. The physician may claim that extending life is "futile" even while conceding it is physiologically possible. The physician is claiming there is no value in the activity while the patient or surrogate has claimed that it is of value. The critical moral claim is that experts in a domain such as medicine can claim no legitimate expertise on these normative judgments. Some physicians see value in permanently unconscious life; most do not — just as some lay people see value in such life while most do not. The dispute cannot be resolved by medical expertise. Ths issue is whether patients, in addition to having a right to refuse medical treatments, also can have a right to access to some treatments even if they are deemed normatively futile by the physician providers. Presumably, some treatments demanded by patients can be resisted by health professionals even if they agree on the physiological outcomes. Some treatments are simply too trivial or too controversial to assume that a patient who has a correct understanding of the physiological effect of the intervention automatically has a right of access from an unwilling provider. Providers can refuse to provide cosmetic surgery, experimental treatments, obesity therapies, and many other kinds of treatments including morally controversial interventions such as abortions or euthanasia. They may claim it is simply not a therapy they choose to offer. (In fact, in some cases they are legally forbidden from offering it.) Even though providers may clearly refuse to provide some classes of treatments, are there certain kinds of treatment patients may justifiably demand? To put the question in other words, are there some classes of treatments that providers may, in good conscience, not refuse to provide?

Resource Allocation and the Ends of Medicine

The American discussion has made a further distinction at this point. When asked why a provider may justifiably refuse to provide a treatment, one obvious reason put forward is the moral imperative to conserve scarce resources. When a treatment achieves only those effects that some would consider to be of no value at all, someone could plausibly ask whether such treatment is a good use of scarce medical resources. All societies face the problem of scarcity of resources and should think carefully about policies to limit their inefficient use.

Why Resource Allocation is Not the Central Issue

Although treatments deemed futile by providers seem to be the epitome of inefficient resource use, there are three reasons why that has not been the main focus of the futility debate. First, as we have suggested, even though a provider may see no value in the effect of some treatment, others (including the patient) may see those effects as valuable. Any policy limiting the use of resources for treatments deemed futile by providers must take into account the subjectivity of judgments about what counts as a valuable treatment effect. Some effects may be seen as being of value by others even if they are deemed valueless by a provider. Hence, there is reason to question the provider's refusal to provide.

Second, even if there is a substantial consensus that the treatment effect is of questionable value, there is reason to hold that someone other than the patient's physician should set limits on the use of medical resources on grounds of responsible use of resources. The physician is, at least historically, committed morally to the welfare of the patient, not the interests of other parties. He or she may at least see psychological benefits to the patient who receives a treatment that is very much desired. In fact, the physician, being historically committed to the patient, may actually over-commit scarce resources to his or her patient if they provide some level of benefit, no matter how inefficient.

Third, even if treatments deemed futile by providers are good candidates to be eliminated in the name of social justice and the fair and efficient use of scarce resources, this class of treatments is not unique in being considered for such limits. Other treatments, admittedly not "futile," may be very inefficient in the benefits they provide for the resources invested or may be very unfair use of resources and may be good candidates to be eliminated in a program designed to address the issues of resource allocation.

Futility and the Ends of Medicine

Although scarcity of resources may often be a justifiable reason to place a limit on any treatment, often the cases identified as "futile care cases" in the American discussion have not raised this issue. It turns out that the cases have not involved scarce resources and that funding for the treatment is available without jeopardizing the welfare of those who have just claims on social resources. Some futile care cases involve settings in which all involved acknowledge no scarcity of hospital facilities or health professional personnel. The funding of the treatment may come from sources for which the patient has a just claim. For example, the patient may have bought special insurance to cover the service, in effect, pre-paying for the treatment deemed futile and not consuming social resources to which the patient is not entitled. Alternatively, the patient may self-pay (ideally using personal resources justly acquired). Or a group sympathetic to the patient's demands may pool resources to pay for the treatment as an act of charity. These could be referred to as "equitable funding sources" in that, in theory, the patient has a legitimate claim on the resource and is not consuming something to which others are justly entitled.

The central moral issue of care deemed futile is whether, independent of resource issues, there are moral arguments unique to this class of treatments that justify a physician's refusal to provide or, alternatively, whether there are arguments that support a patient's right of access.

Often in the American cases, physicians have claimed that they have a new understanding of the ends of medicine to which they are obligated. These ends are often expressed as the "healing of the patient" and are presumed not to include interventions that merely stabilize a dying patient in an unconscious or otherwise seriously compromised state. Physicians opposing care they deem futile hold they have no professional obligation to deliver a service that is outside the ends of medicine. If a patient is to have a right of access to an unwilling physician's services to provide treatments he or she deems futile and outside the ends of medicine, some strong moral argument will be needed.

Autonomy and Access to Futile Care

Some critics of the advocates of access to treatments deemed futile by physicians in the case in which the patient sees an agreed-upon outcome as valuable have argued or assumed that the defense of access is based on some theory of patient autonomy (Paris 1993). At least more sophisticated defenses of patient access to treatments deemed futile by providers do not, however, rest on the ethical principle of autonomy. Autonomy is a principle that largely creates negative rights — the right to refuse treatment, for example. It does not give someone the right to the services of another party. In fact, insofar as autonomy is concerned, it is the autonomy of the provider that is in jeopardy in disputes over futile care. The demand of the patient is that the physician participate in the patient's treatment against the provider's will. Autonomy, if anything, seems to support the right of providers not to participate in delivering care against their professional judgment.

Professional Promises and Access to Futile Care

Hence, if a right of access is to be established, it must rest on other moral grounds. The grounds most often cited in the American discussion has been the health professional's duty growing out of the principle of fidelity or promise keeping. When physicians take on a patient, they generally promise to stay with the patient and serve the patient until relieved of that responsibility either by the patient's agreement or by their replacement by another willing physician. If there is another physician competent to provide the treatment sought by the patient and willing to provide it, both patient and provider would plausibly agree to the substitution of the new health professional. In all the interesting American cases, which will be discussed later, no competent colleague willing to serve could be located.

Some would reply that the health professional's promise to stay with a patient is not open-ended; it applies only to those services within the standard of care. If the treatments deemed futile for the health professional are not in the standard of care, then they are not within the promise of loyalty to the patient. That makes sense and applies to cases of patients demanding physiologically futile treatments as well as treatments that are marginal to medical well-being (such as cosmetic treatments). It does not make sense, however, to exclude certain narrow classes of treatments that have historically been seen as part of the standard duty of the physician.

Drawing on a concept of the law, we can identify a patient's interest in a small class of cases in which we would say the patient's interest is fundamental. This suggests the necessity of differentiating a large group of treatments in which the patient's interest is considered more marginal or controversial — cosmetic procedures, experimental procedures, and controversial interventions such as abortion — from a smaller group of treatments in which a patient might be said to have a basic or fundamental interest. Saving a life with treatments that will effectively prolong life is such an example. Possibly, relief of severe pain would be another such fundamental interest. The claim is that the professional's promise to stay with the patient must include provision of services that serve a fundamental interest of the patient when that service has historically been within the standard of care.

The distinction calls for a mental exercise. Imagine there is a situation in which a majority of the population would not want an intervention (such as life prolongation for patients in a vegetative state) while a minority would have a strong desire for the intervention. Imagine further that one did not know whether one were in the majority or minority. The claim is that for a few treatments, even if we were in the majority, we could empathize with those in the minority to the point that we would support their right of access. We would adopt a policy that is cognizant of the minority's claim and see it as so fundamental that we would not want to risk the possibility that at some point in the future we would be in the minority and have to face a social policy that excluded our right of access. This approach, modeled after the veil of ignorance methodology of twentieth-century American philosopher John Rawls (1971), suggests that basic social policies should be designed so as to treat worse-off minorities in a fair manner.

Historically, physicians have regularly provided life-prolonging treatments, at least if patients desired the treatment (and sometimes even if they did not). The historical pattern in effect amounts to a mutual set of promises between the society and the profession. The profession will be given, as a privilege of licensure, a monopoly on the use of life-sustaining technologies in exchange for which a reasonable society would extract the promise that, under certain specified conditions, a physician will use those technologies on patients who want them. Among the conditions that plausibly would be imposed:

1) The treatment is in the context of an ongoing patient-physician relation.
2) The physician is competent to provide the treatment.
3) No other competent colleague is willing to take the case.
4) Some equitable funding source is available to pay for the treatment.
5) The interest at stake is deemed fundamental (life preserving or pain relieving).

The claim of the defenders of patient access to life-prolonging care deemed futile is that the cases in the American discussion meet all five of these conditions.

RELATED LEGISLATION AND POLICY DEALING WITH MEDICAL FUTILITY

These moral arguments for the patient's limited right of access to care deemed futile by providers emerged in the 1990s through case law in the American courts and limited legislative efforts at the state level.

Case Law

Several legal cases generally led to the conclusion that, when the five conditions we have identified were present, the patient had a right of access. These cases were often settled on various technical legal grounds but all supported the patient's right of access.

Helga Wanglie (1989–1991)

The first case gaining widespread public attention was that of Helga Wanglie (*In re The Conservatorship of Helga Wanglie* 1991). Mrs. Wanglie had suffered a hip fracture in December of 1989. While being transferred from a nursing home to the Hennepin County Medical Center by ambulance on January 1, 1990, she suffered a cardiac arrest. This was followed by other cardiac arrests, including one on May 23, 1990, which left her in a state of unconsciousness from which she did not recover. She was left ventilator-dependent and was fed only by intubation. At this point she had aortic insufficiency, congestive heart failure, chronic, recurrent pneumonias, and chronic respiratory insufficiency. She was in a persistent vegetative state from which her physicians concluded she would never recover.

There had been various reports that Mrs. Wanglie and her husband of 53 years, Oliver, were devout Lutherans with "pro-life" views. Mr. Wanglie, in consultation with their son and daughter, insisted that ventilator support continue. Consultation with the hospital ethics committee led to the recommendation that Mrs. Wanglie's ventilator be removed, a recommendation which Mr. Wanglie refused to accept.

Steven H. Miles, a member of the committee and consultant to the physicians treating Mrs. Wanglie, sought to have Mr. Wanglie removed as decision-maker for his wife. The working assumption was that the removal of Mr. Wanglie and appointment of a new guardian would lead to a decision to remove the ventilator, which the medical personnel deemed futile.

The court found that Mr. Wanglie was his wife's closest relative, knew her conscientious, religious, and moral beliefs, had a well-established pattern of conferring with family members, and was dedicated to promoting his wife's welfare. It thus confirmed the appointment of him as her guardian and denied Steven Miles's counter-effort. The decision, while technically only a guardian determination, was widely interpreted as an affirmation of the right of Mr. Wanglie to insist on continued life support for his wife. She died on July 4, 1991, six days after the court decision. Her medical costs of $800,000 were paid primarily by Medicare and a supplemental insurer. Only a small portion of the costs arose after the court decision.

Baby K (1992–1994)

On October 13, 1992, a baby was born in Virginia, widely referred to as "Baby K," who had been diagnosed prenatally as having anencephaly. The mother insisted that life support be continued. The physicians, with the advice of the hospital's ethics committee, believed that ventilatory support was not warranted and sought legal authority in the federal court to forgo it. The court, summarizing the baby's condition, described her as lacking a cerebrum and, hence, permanently unconscious (*In the Matter of Baby K* 1993). She had no cognitive abilities or awareness and could not hear or otherwise interact with her environment. At birth, physicians placed the baby on a mechanical ventilator, confirmed the diagnosis, and recommended the baby be supplied with nutrition, hydration, and warmth, but that no aggressive treatment be provided. Baby K's mother continued to insist on mechanical breathing assistance.

Attorneys for the mother argued that American laws required provision of assistance. They appealed to the Emergency Medical Treatment and Active Labor Act (EMTALA), which requires hospitals to provide emergency treatment of all patients, as well as the Rehabilitation Act, which prohibits discrimination against the handicapped, and Americans with Disabilities Act as well as other federal and state laws. The court ruled that, based on these laws, the hospital had to provide ventilator treatment to Baby K. The decision was appealed to the United States Court of Appeals, which upheld the decision (*In the Matter of Baby K* 1994). When an appeal was made to the United States Supreme Court, that court declined to hear the case, thus upholding the ruling.

It is important to this case that Baby K's mother did not challenge any of the medical facts of the case as presented by the attorneys for the hospital. She acknowledged that the baby had true anencephaly and would never recover consciousness. Nevertheless, she disagreed with the physicians' value judgment that there was no value in preserving the unconscious life. This was, thus, a dispute over normative, not physiological, futility. Baby K, from the point of the decision, continued to receive high-quality medical care and survived for two and a half years before succumbing to an infection.

Other Cases in Which Treatment was Required

Since the time of Helga Wanglie and Baby K almost all other reported cases involving futility have led to legal decisions that life support must be required. They generally involved normative controversies in which physicians and patients or families agreed on the likely therapeutic outcome of intervention. Generally, they were cases in which the patient's condition would not be cured and the patient would not be restored to consciousness. The disputes have generally been over whether unconscious life was worth preserving. With a limited number of exceptions described later, these cases are now usually not formally debated. Patients are presumed to have the right of access to life-sustaining medical interventions, regardless of the opinion of physicians that the treatment outcome is not worth pursuing.

In a case in the state of Georgia, a doctor allowed a premature baby to die by terminating life support against the wishes of the parents. The Court of Appeals of Georgia ruled that the doctor "had no right to decide, unilaterally, to discontinue medical treatment even if, as the record in this case reflects, the child was terminally ill and in the process of dying. That decision must be made with the consent of the parents" (*Velez* v. *Bethune et al.* 1995). That court cited an earlier Georgia court opinion with similar implications (*In re Jane Doe, a minor* 1991; *In re Doe* 1992). Similar results were reported from a lower court case in Pennsylvania (*Rideout, Administrator of Estate of Rideout, et al.* v. *Hershey Medical Center* 1995).

A Single Legal Case with Contrary Implications: Catherine Gilgunn (1989–1995)

In the face of this rather consistent legal history of courts ruling that physicians did not have the authority to unilaterally forgo life-sustaining medical treatment without patient or surrogate approval, one court case seems to have contrary implications. It is the nature of United States laws that many cases are decided by state rather than federal courts, and they may be governed by somewhat different laws. The single case seeming to be consistent with the right of physicians to forgo unilaterally treatments they believe to be futile arises in Massachusetts. It presents unusual details, making it difficult to determine whether the Massachusetts courts would have supported the physicians' decisions to forgo care they deemed futile in any of the other cases described earlier.

In May of 1989 a 72-year-old woman named Catherine Gilgunn broke her hip. (The legal opinion resulting from this case was unpublished. This summary is based on Kolata 1995a, 1995b; Paris *et al.* 1999; Orr 1999; Zucker 1995; Capron 1995.) She had a previous history of diabetes, kidney problems, coronary artery disease, breast cancer, and Parkinsonism, as well as three previous hip replacements. After she initially refused treatment, her daughter, who was her primary caregiver, called an ambulance. Before the surgery could take place, she had several seizures. She could only manifest grimacing and withdrawal. Her prospects for recovery were described as dismal. At this point the attending physician recommended a decision not to resuscitate in the event of a cardiac arrest, often called a do-not-resuscitate (DNR) order.

Other family members agreed that the daughter was the patient's proper spokesperson. She rejected the DNR order. Upon consultation with the hospital's ethics committee, the chair of the committee indicated that resuscitation would be "a violation of standard practices for this patient" (Paris *et al.* 1999, p. 42). A DNR order initially placed was rescinded at the insistence of the daughter. After many more days of further medical complications and deterioration, the ethics committee once again recommended the placing of the DNR order, which was the course followed by the attending. The attending informed the family and began the process of weaning the patient from the ventilator. The patient died on August 10, 1989. The case led the family to bring charges against the physician. After a trial in the Superior Court of Massachusetts, the court ruled on April 22, 1995, that the charges were not sustained (Kolata 1995a). The decision was widely regarded as finding that the physician need not provide treatment that he or she deems futile even if the family insists. The exact meaning of the decision, however, is hard to determine since there was no opinion published by the court. If the finding was that the physician need not deliver such care, it conflicts with all the previous cases mentioned. There are several other possibilities, however. Noting that Mrs. Gilgunn initially refused treatment, some have suggested that perhaps the judge concluded that, contrary to her daughter's stated view, Mrs. Gilgunn really did not want the resuscitation. That, of course, would not only permit the physician to withhold, but would require it. Others have noticed the ambiguity in the physician's language describing CPR as "medically contraindicated" as well as "inhumane and unethical." There is some suggestion that the daughter continued to believe that the resuscitation could be successful while the physician's reference to contraindication might suggest his belief that it literally could not succeed in restarting her heart. In that case, this could be a dispute over whether CPR was physiologically futile, an issue over which we have suggested physicians legitimately claim authority. On the other hand, claiming CPR was "inhumane and unethical" seems to suggest a dispute not over whether CPR could at least temporarily succeed in restarting her heart, but rather whether the pain and suffering CPR would cause would be worth it — an issue of normative dispute. Still others have pointed out that this case is unique in attempting to prosecute long after the death of the patient a physician who unilaterally withdrew treatment. It seems there is little the court could do at this point. By contrast the other futile care cases have addressed decisions while the patient was still alive and physicians were seeking authority to act unilaterally. Whatever the explanation of the decision, some analysts have criticized the finding (Capron 1995) and it conflicts with all the other US legal cases if it exonerates the physicians.

State Futility Policies

In contrast with the case law, which, with this one exception, has supported the right of patients and families to have access to treatments deemed futile by their physicians provided the five conditions mentioned before are met, two states of the United States have attempted to speak to the issue of futility through legislative and regulatory approaches, both appearing to carve out a set of circumstances under which a physician could unilaterally withhold or withdraw treatments that are sustaining life even though the patient or family objected to such action.

Texas and Virginia have adopted such policies. The Texas policy was, by statute, incorporated into the Texas Advance Directives Act in 1999 and has become part of the Texas Health and Safety Code (1999). Virginia's policy is substantially similar in spite of the fact that the Baby K case led to federal court decisions requiring at least emergency treatment in that state. Section 166.052 of the Texas Health and Safety Code sets out circumstances under which a physician may unilaterally withhold or withdraw life-sustaining treatment against the wishes of the patient or surrogates. If the physician considers the requested life-sustaining procedure to be "inappropriate," the patient or surrogate is to be given 48 hours' notice that a committee will review the case and is entitled to attend the meeting. If the committee concurs that the treatment is inappropriate, the physician, with the help of the facility, must assist the patient in trying to find a facility willing to provide the requested treatment. In the meantime, the patient is to be given the requested treatment for up to 10 days. The key sentence reads, "If a provider cannot be found willing to give the requested treatment within 10 days, life-sustaining treatment may be withdrawn unless a court of law has granted an extension" (Code of Virginia, Title 54.1, Professions and Occupations, 54.1–2990). In other words, Texas law authorizes a process whereby physicians may unilaterally withdraw or withhold life support from patients who, in some cases, could live with treatment (at least for a while) even though the patients or their surrogates desperately want their life to continue. Virginia law does not require referral to a committee and allows the patient 14 days to find an alternative caregiver.

Given that this is a public, governmental policy growing out of legislation, it lacks some of the sophistication of the more nuanced discussion. For example, no distinction is made between physiological and normative futility. The physician must merely find the treatment "inappropriate." The policy has also been criticized because it leaves very sick and vulnerable patients or their surrogates with the responsibility of finding alternative facilities willing to take their cases within 10 days.

Two cases have received considerable publicity related to this futility policy. The earliest case involves an infant named Sun Hudson (based on Veatch 2005; Hopper 2005. Note that there was some systematic confusion regarding the infant's first name. It was widely noted his mother named him with a religious reference in mind. Some, in what now appears to be an error, used the name "Son" (as in Son of God) while others, correctly, used the name "Sun" (as a reference to the Sun god).). Sun was born on September 25, 2004, with a form of dwarfism and had lungs too small to sustain life. The father was unknown. The mother, Wanda Hudson, apparently suggested the boy's father was the Sun, hence his name. Physicians at Texas Children's Hospital in Houston invoked the provisions of the Texas Health and Safety Code that permitted unilateral withdrawal of life support against the wishes of the mother, who protested. After the 10-day waiting period and some further delay involving legal complications, the physicians withdrew the tube supporting respiration. He died on March 15, 2005, within a minute of the removal of the tube.

The Texas law, like other ambiguous futility policies, authorizes removal of life support by a physician when the physician (with the concurrence of a committee) finds the treatment "inappropriate," thus failing to distinguish claims based in medical science that the treatment will not accomplish the intended purpose, from claims based in evaluative judgments that the treatment's effects are not sufficiently valuable. The fact that Sun Hudson lived for six months, while the provisions of the Act were executed, makes clear that the respiratory support was effective in preserving life, at least in the short run. The case against Sun Hudson's treatment was either that such a life was of no value or that the pain he endured was not worth it. In addition to the controversy over the use of the Texas legal provision, the case posed additional problems. There were suggestions that some doubted the mother's mental competence to act as her son's decision-maker. Given the concern expressed about the suffering of the child, it is possible that this case should have been handled not as a futile care case, but rather as one involving a parent (like a Jehovah's Witness parent refusing blood) who makes a seriously inappropriate decision about what is in her child's best interest. The medical personnel could have followed the route of seeking to have her removed from the guardian role on grounds of competence and had a court-appointed guardian make a best interest determination. If serious, needless suffering resulted from the life support, the guardian may have decided to forgo further support.

A number of other cases of unilateral treatment withdrawal have been reported based on the Texas Advance Directives Act. Since the law does not require reporting such decisions it is impossible to know the number. One report indicates at least 27 cases have occurred.

Many have noted a striking and problematic dimension of this case and its relation to the case of Terri Schiavo, the Florida woman maintained for many years in a vegetative state while various courts and government agencies attempted to determine the proper decision-making procedures for her care. In the Schiavo case, early courts (eventually sustained) decided, based on testimony from her husband and others, that she would want artificial nutrition and hydration removed so she could be allowed to die. This was criticized by her parents, advocates for pro-life perspectives (including some in the Catholic church), and eventually US President George W. Bush, on the grounds that public policy should support life in such cases. According to these critics, the courts and public figures should not make use of the government apparatus to make decisions leading to withdrawal of life support and the death of an incompetent and vulnerable patient.

By contrast, the Texas Advance Directives Act futility provisions use public policy adopted through state law to authorize ending the lives of similarly vulnerable, incompetent patients even against the wishes of their parents or guardians. The striking thing is that the Texas policy was signed into law by the then governor of Texas, one George W. Bush.

Recently, efforts have been launched by pro-life advocates as well as defenders of patients' rights to repeal or modify the Texas Advance Directives Act provisions authorizing unilateral forgoing of life support against the wishes of patients and their surrogates. An amendment was introduced into the 2007 legislative session that would have changed the law to require that life support demanded by patients or family be continued until a patient can be transferred. The proposed law was called the Patient and Family Treatment Choice Rights Act of 2007. The bill was passed by the Texas State Senate, but was not acted upon in the House. In subsequent years, further efforts to amend or repeal the law have been attempted without success.

HOW DECISIONS ARE MADE IN THE CASE OF FUTILE CARE AND BY WHOM — PHYSICIAN? FAMILY MEMBERS? OR TOGETHER?

As can be seen by this review, the debate in the United States over decisions to withhold or withdraw treatments deemed futile by the physician represents a shifting scene. As recently as the 1980s, some physicians in the United States still insisted that they had the sole responsibility for medical decisions and that their role as physician required first, and foremost, that they make decisions that would preserve human life whenever possible. Hence, most physicians never faced the problem of deciding to withdraw futile care that could effectively affect the dying trajectory of the patient. If an intervention could preserve life, even briefly and even with burden to the patient, that intervention was required. Patients, beginning in the 1960s and 1970s, began to fight for the right to make decisions to refuse such life-extending interventions when they believed the burden of the treatment outweighed the benefits. In these choices they were supported not only by secular liberals and Protestants, but also by Roman Catholics who had long endorsed a doctrine of extraordinary means that accepted refusal of treatments that were, on balance, burdensome. Some Orthodox Jews and some other groups generally too small to make an impact on the public consciousness agreed with physicians that life should always be preserved when possible, but lay people generally led the fight to change public policy.

Very soon physicians joined the "death with dignity" movement and began to articulate the view that preserving life in an unconscious or seriously compromised state was not always worth it. Some physicians even began to claim that such preservation was inconsistent with the ends of medicine and that they had a moral duty to resist. This left minority groups of patients — some pro-life Catholics and Protestants, as well as some Jews and Muslims — dissenting from the new consensus and insisting that life-supporting treatments be provided as long as certain conditions were met. If the treatment would effectively extend life (even briefly), was being considered in an ongoing doctor-patient relation in which the doctor was competent to deliver the life-extending intervention, was equitably funded, and served a fundamental interest of the patient, patients from these minority perspectives increasingly insisted on their right of access. In this they were supported by some patients' rights advo-cates, even those who had earlier led the fight to get physicians to stop imposing life support against a patient's wishes. Since the vigorous debate of the 1990s we are now in a more quiescent period where most seem to assume that the advocates for patients and surrogates who want treatments deemed futile by their physicians should have a right of access provided the specified conditions are met. That has been the result of almost all court cases. The major exception is in the states of Texas and Virginia where unusual and controversial laws are still being debated. In general, in the United States federal laws prevail over state laws so one can assume that the federal decisions in the Baby K case that grant a right to at least emergency life-prolonging treatment are established even if a more general access to treatments deemed futile is still debated at least in these two states.

HOW THE ISSUE OF MEDICAL FUTILITY IS DISTINGUISHED FROM EUTHANASIA

In the United States the debate over medical futility has largely occurred independent of the debate over euthanasia. This is in part because eutha-nasia — defined as the intentional action to end a person's life on the grounds that the burdens are overwhelming — is sharply distinguished from the patient's right to forgo life support. While the former is generally illegal (assisted suicide in Oregon, Washington, and Montana being the exception), the right to refuse life support is now clearly established legally and most people accept it ethically.

The debate over medical futility is seen as a corollary of the patient's right to forgo life support. The complicating feature is that a right of access to treatments deemed futile by physicians requires the cooperation of those physicians when professional autonomy has generally been the norm. Forgoing life support requires only that the physician step aside; granting access to treatments deemed futile requires the physician's active participation. Hence, the right of access cannot effectively be based on the ethical principle of autonomy. It must rest on a duty of the professional which has best been grounded in promises made as part of the establish-ment of the monopoly privileges of licensure. If patients forswear the right to use life-prolonging medical technologies themselves, they must reserve the right to get access to those technologies in cases in which they want them and only licensed professionals are permitted to provide them. Hence, even though professionals, like lay people, generally have an autonomy right to control their own actions, they are seen as surrendering that right as part of the establishment of the general social practice of medicine. Just as physicians promise not to violate laws governing narcotics if they are to be accepted practitioners, so physicians promise to use technologies that effectively preserve people's lives when patients want them preserved and some carefully defined conditions are met.

FUTURE TRENDS AND DEVELOPMENT

Thus, the debate over medical futility in the United States has matured, but has not been fully resolved. There is probably less debate over the topic than there was in the 1990s, in large part because of the near-consensus in the legal cases that patients and their authorized surrogates have the authority to insist on continued life support in cases in which physicians have claimed normative futility provided certain conditions are met, including the legitimate claim that a desired intervention can produce an effect sought by the patient or patient representative when the physician's reason for wanting to stop is not grounded in resource issues.

The most conspicuous unresolved problem is the law in the state of Texas (and to a lesser extent in Virginia), which seems to authorize limited cases of unilateral refusal of life support even though the patient or patient representative can plausibly claim that the desired effect can be accomplished by medical intervention and a funding source is available to cover the treatment. The paradox is that Texas is a state in which many assertive advocates of the preservation of human life, when possible, voice their "pro-life" views. It seems certain that the law must be clarified so that so-called futile care that can really achieve the patient-centered objective must be provided if no resource constraints are presented. It seems likely that a coalition of those who are inherently "pro-life" and those who defend the right of patients to their own choices will form and prevail. This will still not address the much more complicated question of the right of access to medical care when resources really are at issue. That question will be wrapped up with the current debate over the Affordable Care Act, the Obama administration's effort to provide near-universal health insurance, which is so strongly opposed by conservative private property advocates, but which was recently affirmed by the United States Supreme Court.

REFERENCES

Capron AM. 1995. Abandoning a waning life [Catherine Gilgunn]. *The Hastings Center Report* 25: 24–26.

Code of Virginia, Title 54.1, Professions and Occupations, 54.1–2990.

Council on Ethical and Judicial Affairs, American Medical Association. 1999. Medical futility in end-of-life care. *Journal of the American Medical Association* 281: 937–941.

Hopper L. 2005. Baby born with fatal defect dies after removal from life support. *Houston Chronicle*, March 15. Available at: http://www.chron.com/news/houstontexas/article/Baby-born-with-fatal-defect-dies-after-removal-1498268.php [Accessed March 1, 2012].

In re Doe, 418 S.E.2d 3 (Ga. 1992).

In re Jane Doe, a minor, Civil Action File No. D-93064, Superior Court of Fulton County, State of Georgia, October 1991.

In re The Conservatorship of Helga Wanglie, State of Minnesota, District Court, Probate Court Division, County of Hennepin, Fourth Judicial District, June 28, 1991.

In the Matter of Baby K, 832 F.Supp. 1022 (E.D. Va. 1993).

In the Matter of Baby K, 16 F.3d 590 (4th Cir. 1994).

Jecker NS and Schneiderman LJ. 1993. Medical futility: The duty not to treat. *Cambridge Quarterly of Healthcare Ethics* 2: 151–159.

Kolata G. 1995a. Court ruling limits rights of patients: Care deemed futile may be withheld. *New York Times*, April 22, p. 6.

Kolata G. 1995b. Withholding care from patients: Boston case asks who decides. *New York Times*, April 3, pp. A1, B8.

Lantos JD, Miles SH, Silverstein MD, and Stocking CB. 1988. Survival after cardiopulmonary resuscitation in babies of very low birth weight: Is CPR futile therapy? *The New England Journal of Medicine* 318: 91–95.

Lantos JD, Singer PA, Walker RM *et al.* 1989. The illusion of futility in clinical practice. *The American Journal of Medicine* 87: 81–84.

Newman R. 2012. One key sector that's still shedding jobs. *US News & World Report*, February 3. Available at: http://news.yahoo.com/one-key-sector-thats-still-shedding-jobs-181314915.html [Accessed February 3, 2012].

Orr RD. 1999. The Gilgunn case: Courage and questions [editorial]. *Journal of Intensive Care Medicine* 14: 54–56.

Paris JJ. 1993. Pipes, colanders, and leaky buckets: Reflections on the futility debate. *Cambridge Quarterly for Healthcare Ethics* 2: 147–149.

Paris JJ, Cassem EH, Dec GW, and Reardon FE. 1999. Use of a DNR order over family objections: The case of Gilgunn v. MGH. *Journal of Intensive Care Medicine* 14: 41–45.

President's Commission for the Study of Ethical Problems in Medicine and Biomedical and Behavioral Research. 1983. *Deciding to Forego Life-Sustaining Treatment: Ethical, Medical, and Legal Issues in Treatment Decisions*. Washington, DC: US Government Printing Office.

Rawls J. 1971. *A Theory of Justice*. Cambridge, MA: Harvard University Press.

Rideout, Administrator of Estate of Rideout, et al. v. *Hershey Medical Center*, Dauphin County Report, 1995, pp. 472–498.

Rubin SB. 1998. *When Doctors Say No: The Battleground of Medical Futility*. Bloomington, IN: Indiana University Press.

Schneiderman LJ, Jecker NS, and Jonsen AR. 1990. Medical futility: Its meaning and ethical implications. *Annals of Internal Medicine* 112: 949–954.

Texas Health & Safety Code, Chapter 166, Subchapter A, §166.046 and 52, 1999.

Velez v. *Bethune et al.*, 466 S.E. 2d 627 (Ga. App. 1995).

Veatch RM. 1973. Generalization of expertise: Scientific expertise and value judgments. *Hastings Center Studies* 1: 29–40.

Veatch RM. 2005. Terri Schiavo, Son Hudson, and 'nonbeneficial' medical treatments. *Health Affairs* 24: 976–979.

Veatch RM. 2009. The evolution of death and dying controversies. *The Hastings Center Report* 39: 16–19.

Veatch RM and Spicer CM. 1992. Medically futile care: The role of the physician in setting limits. *American Journal of Law & Medicine* 18: 15–36.

Youngner SJ. 1988. Who defines futility? *Journal of the American Medical Association* 260: 2094–2095.

Youngner SJ. 1990. Futility in context. *Journal of the American Medical Association* 264: 1295–1296.

Zucker A. 1995. Law and ethics: Withholding care: A test case [Catherine Gilgunn]. *Death Studies* 19: 521–525.

CHAPTER TWO

THE REALITY OF MEDICAL FUTILITY
(DYSTHANASIA) IN BRAZIL

Leo Pessini and William Saad Hossne

SUMMARY

The ethical discussions of end-of-life issues are still somewhat considered a taboo in many countries of Latin America, including Brazil. Little by little with the introduction of bioethics in the curriculum of the healthcare professionals, this situation is changing. This article presents the state of the art related to the issue of medical futility or *dysthanasia* in Brazil. To explore the issue of medical futility in Brazil, this article presents the healthcare system in Brazil, the issues related to end of life in Brazil, some information about ICUs, do-not-resuscitate (DNR) orders and advance directives as well as ethical-juridical discussions about life-sustaining treatment. In doing so, the Brazilian code of ethics and the new Code of Medical Ethics will be discussed. The issue of palliative care as related to futility decision making also will be discussed.

INTRODUCTION

In Brazil, the concept of *dysthanasia* corresponds to therapeutic obstinacy or withdrawal of treatment in end-of-life care. The term "futile treatment" is more used in Anglo-Saxon countries, especially in the United States, England, Australia and other English-speaking countries (Schneiderman 2008; Cassel 1991). Therapeutic obstinacy, in its turn, is the nomenclature adopted by the European countries and originates from the French *l'acharnement thérapeutique*, an expression that arose in the 1950s. In Brazil, the concept of medical futility is known as dysthanasia, which occurs when we fail to recognize that a medical intervention or a medical treatment is futile. By recognizing futile treatments, physicians can step back and avoid relentlessly pursuing the *cure*, where only *care* is applicable and necessary. Therefore, in this scenario, in dealing with medical futility, palliative medicine needs to be introduced.

The obsession with maintaining biological life at any cost leads us to therapeutic obstinacy, or dysthanasia. In this context, the instruments, which in principle are used for cure and care, are transformed into tools of torture, imprisoning the patient amid tubes and appliances that do not do any kind of good but just prolong a painful process of dying, treating death as if it were a disease for which physicians must find a cure! We must not forget that mortality is a dimension of our existence and that death is a natural part of our life and medical investments or treatment at the end of life must have a limit (Schneiderman 2008; Pessini 2005). The concept of *orthothanasia* that was popularized in Brazil in the last decade by some bioethicists and the media is being used to differentiate actions that would be promoting euthanasia, as well as actions that would be promoting dysthanasia. Orthothanasia means by its philological roots (Latin) "death in the right place and time" or "good death". It's situated between two extremes. On one hand not to shorten the life of a patient, which would be euthanasia. And on the other hand not to prolong the long and painful process of dying, which would be dysthanasia. It should be noted that the concept of orthothanasia used here is the same as that of good death in the Anglo-Saxon culture (Pessini *et al.* 2010; Martin 1993, 1999).

THE BRAZILIAN HEALTHCARE SYSTEM

According to the Brazilian Institute of Geography and Statistics (2010), Brazil today has a population of 194 million inhabitants. Since 1988, with the new Brazilian Constitution's enactment, "the right to health for all" has been proclaimed. With the new Federal Constitution, a radical transformation in the Brazilian healthcare system has occurred. The healthcare system assumes a universalist dimension, with health becoming the right of all Brazilian citizens, independent of them being formal workers or not (Fortes 2012).

Article 196 of the Constitution states: "Health is a right of all and a duty of the State, guaranteed by means of social and economic policies aimed at reducing the risk of illness and other hazards and at providing universal and egalitarian access to actions and services for its promotion, protection, and recovery."

In order to make the right to health a reality, the Single Health System (SUS) was organized, with the following guidelines: (1) decentralization, with a single direction in each sphere of government, (2) full assistance, with priority for preventive activities, without prejudice to assistance services, and (3) community participation.

Today the SUS is considered the largest public health system in the world, assisting approximately 150 million Brazilians from the poorer classes. Around 48 million Brazilians who have better life conditions, those in the middle and upper class, have private health and insurance plans. The SUS has currently over 55,000 health institutions, federal, state, and local institutions, and a private philanthropic and charitable network providing services through conventions with the SUS.

The budget for the Ministry of Health for 2011 was approximately US$48 billion (68.8 billion reais), an amount considered still insufficient to meet all the needs of the population. The SUS is the only alternative for 78% of the Brazilian population. The expenditure on health in Brazil represents 8.4% of the GDP. Out of this total, 58.4% was spent by families, while 41.6% by the public sector. In the developed countries, 70% of disbursements are covered by the government, and only 30% by the families. In the country there are almost 432,000 hospital beds, 152,800 of which (35.4%) are public and 279,100 (64.6%) belong to private and philanthropic hospitals. The child mortality rate in 2010 was 19.88 deaths per 1,000 live births. The average life expectancy of Brazilians reached almost 73 years.

In Brazil there are 186 colleges of medicine and 371,786 physicians. According to the World Health Organization, it has much more than necessary to meet the population's needs, but there is an unequal and unfair distribution of physicians, with the majority prevalence in the country's southeastern and southern regions, and a shortage of medical professionals in the northern and northeastern regions.

The Brazilian Association of Intensive Medicine (AMIB) prepared in 2009 the first study intended at presenting a view of the scenario of intensive care units (ICUs) in the country, the AMIB Census. In terms of intensive medicine in Brazil, there are 2,342 ICUs with 25,367 ICU beds in 1,421 health institutions. Of these ICUs, adult ICUs make up 89%, neonatal ICUs 30.2%, children ICUs 19.7% and 0.6% of ICUs are for patients with burns.

It should be mentioned that 25.2% of these ICUs belong to the public sector, 39.5% to the private sector and 33.5% to charitable/philanthropic organizations.

According to the Ministry of Health (Directive no. 1101/CM, June 12, 2001) we have the following assistance cover parameters in terms of hospital beds, which is estimated as follows: For total hospital beds, from 2.5 to 3 beds for every 1,000 inhabitants. For ICU beds, it is calculated, on average, that 4% to 10% of total hospital beds are needed. This corresponds to 1 to 3 ICU beds for every 10,000 inhabitants. The Brazilian average is 1.3 ICU beds for every 10,000 inhabitants. As observed in relation to the number of health institutions, health professionals, hospital and ICU bed numbers, the southeast and south of Brazil are well, while in other Brazilian regions almost everything is missing (AMIB 2009).

END-OF-LIFE ISSUES AND THE CODE OF MEDICAL ETHICS IN BRAZIL

In Brazil, dealing with end-of-life issues is based on the Code of Medical Ethics which has been revised several times.

Brazil approved a new Code of Medical Ethics which became effective on April 13, 2010. This achievement results from a long reflection and revision process of the Code of 1988, led by the National Revision

Commission of the Code of Medical Ethics with broad public participation. Our reflection is grounded in the study of the historic tradition of the
Brazilian Code of Medical Ethics.

In 2007, the Federal Council of Medicine (CFM), which is the highest
authority in the country regulating the professional exercise of the 371,786
physicians (December 2011) who work in Brazil, revised the previous
(1988) Code of Medical Ethics.

After 22 years, many things have changed in Brazil, especially in the
healthcare area, in terms of citizen awareness about the "right to health"
and also the ethical behavior of the population and healthcare professionals. The country has experienced a true technological revolution, which
has had a profound effect on human life, from before birth to after an
individual is declared dead. We are entering the age of genomics medicine, telemedicine, medically assisted reproduction and nanotechnology,
to name just a few novelties. These are some of the factors that create a
new scenario in the healthcare system which requires bioethical reflection, a new ethical awareness and ethical guidelines.

In Brazil, in a period of nearly a century and a half, more precisely 145
years (1867–2012), nine codes of ethics have been introduced. These
codes are the first Code of Medical Ethics which was a translation of the
Code of Medical Ethics of the American Medical Association of 1867;
then the Code of Medical Morality in 1929; the Code of Medical
Deontology in 1931, 1945 and 1984; the Code of Ethics of the Brazilian
Medical Association in 1953; the Code of Medical Ethics in 1965 and
1988. The most recent one, the Code of Medical Ethics, approved on
August 29, 2009, became effective on April 13, 2010 (Martin 1993, 1996,
1999; Bertachini and Pessini 2011).

In a historical analysis of the evolution of the discussions about end-of-
life issues in Brazil we will begin with the Code of Medical Deontology
of 1945. The word "death" did not exist in that code. There is a discreet
reference to "death certificates" (Article 35.1.f/1945). In Article 56/1945,
there is a veiled reference to the terminal patient, in which the physicians
are obliged to notify, in certain cases, those who must know, the possibility of complications or a fatal outcome. However, it should be noted that,
accordingly, physicians decide how much information the patient must
have about his health condition, and not the patient. This shows how our

medical system is a paternalistic one, because everything depends on the doctor's judgment (Martin 1993, p. 74).

The doctor-patient relationship is marked by benign paternalism. That Code also mentions what physicians are not allowed, which is "abandoning chronic or incurable cases, without proven reason of force majeure" (Article 4.1.1945). This Article is a revised version of the Code of 1929, which states: "The doctor shall never abandon chronic and incurable cases, and in difficult and prolonged cases it is necessary to hold conferences with other colleagues" (Article 8/1929). In this regard the Code of 1931 states: "The doctor shall never abandon chronic or incurable cases; and in difficult and prolonged cases it will be necessary and perhaps convenient to hold conferences with other colleagues" (Article 8/1931).

Another important provision of the Code of 1945 is related to the management of pain and suffering. In this Code, it is stated that it is the doctor's duty "to make use of the resources within their reach to alleviate those who suffer" (Article 3.5/1945). The Code does not provide any positive hint as to how to proceed. It offers a negative hint by indicating a path not to be followed: the option for euthanasia. The prohibition is absolute: "The doctor is prohibited from advising or practicing euthanasia" (Article 4.5/1945). The Code of 1931 rejects euthanasia, but indicates the need of alleviating pain without taking this "to the extreme of giving death by mercy" (Article 16/1931). The Code of 1929 does not make any reference to euthanasia. The only time the term "euthanasia" arises in the Brazilian codes of medical ethics is in the Code of 1945 (Article 4.5/1945).

Another right of the terminal patient protected by the Code of 1953 is the right of not being abandoned by the doctor. Article 32.a/1953 reinforces Article 4.1/1945 and provides that the doctor cannot "abandon the patient, even in chronic or incurable cases, except due to an irremovable impediment, which should be communicated to the patient or their responsible party with the necessary advice". This Code is important, as it is an implicit recognition that the doctor's role goes beyond the function of curing. It is part of the doctor's actions to follow up and take care of the patient, even when facing a situation of impossibility to cure.

The Code of 1953 brings a novelty in relation to the previous codes as to the value of human life. It provides that it is the doctor's duty "to keep absolute respect for human life, never using the technical or scientific knowledge to impose pain or provoke men's extermination". The Code of 1965 reaffirms this doctor's duty practically with the same words. The Code of 1953 deals with the need of alleviating and taking care of the patient's pain, as well as of the latter's right of not being killed. "The doctor has the duty of doing everything to alleviate the suffering of their patient; however, the doctor will never resort to the excess of contributing, by action or advice, to anticipate the patient's death" (Article 56/1953). The patient's wellness requires that the pain be alleviated and that the life must not be shortened by medical action.

Article 56/1953 represents an irresolvable dilemma for the doctor who wants to sedate the patient with the aim of alleviating pain, but is aware that this procedure will almost certainly have the side effect of shortening the patient's life. On the one hand, the text is emphatic in saying that the doctor "has the duty of doing everything" for the suffering of their patient to be alleviated, but, on the other hand, any action or advice that advances death is rejected. The Code seems to suggest a hierarchy of values pursuant to which the "alleviation of suffering" has precedence over the "absolute respect for life".

The Code of Medical Ethics of 1965 alters this hierarchy by establishing, in Article 57/1965, that "The doctor cannot contribute, either directly or indirectly, to accelerate the patient's death". When prioritizing the absolute respect for life, the text leaves pain alleviation in the background, and, besides, it prohibits not only any direct action, but also any indirect actions that might accelerate death.

The Code of Deontology of 1984, as in the previous codes, approaches the continuing stress between the effort of not causing unnecessary pain to the terminal patient and an injunction that seems to oblige the doctor to use all available resources in order to avoid the patient's death (Article 1/1984). However, the emphasis on alleviating pain and suffering and the emphasis on not accelerating the patient's death continue side by side without indication of how to solve the ethical conflict between the requirements of both. Article 29/1984 prohibits doctors from "contributing to accelerate the patient's death or using artificial means, when brain death is proven". Although a new concept of brain death is introduced based on the technical-scientific evolution of medicine, and there are a lot of ethical discussions around that, it does not clarify, let alone define, its meaning. However, it is important to mention that the concept of brain death appeared for the first time in the Code of 1984, although the issue had already been discussed within the medical sphere since it arose in 1968 with the Harvard definition.

The Code of Medical Ethics of 1988 reinforces the patient's right of not going through a futile treatment. Article 60/1988, with its prohibition of "complicating the therapeutics", reiterates Article 23/1984. Another concern expressed in this Code is the regulation of medical research on terminal patients. Article 130/1988 prohibits the doctor from "carrying out experiments with new clinical or surgical treatments in patients with incurable or terminal illnesses if there is not any reasonable hope for them, not imposing additional sufferings on them". In a quick view of the Code of Medical Ethics of 1988 in relation to the end-of-life issues, 20 years having passed since its approval, it can immediately be noticed that we lived in a social, historic, cultural context of denying human finitude. It does not mention the end of life and how to guide healthcare providers to deal with death in an ethical manner. At most, the doctor is instructed how to act in the face of "imminent life danger" (Articles 46, 56). Article 60 establishes that doctors are prohibited from "exaggerating the diagnosis or prognostic seriousness, complicating the therapeutic". Article 61, paragraph 2, provides that "the doctors cannot abandon the patients because they bear a chronic or incurable illness, but shall continue assisting them, even if only to mitigate physical or psychic suffering". Article 66 prohibits doctors from "using, in any case, any means intended to abbreviate the patient's life, even upon their request or upon request of his legal representative". Although the word "euthanasia" is not employed, this is the issue at stake. The tradition of the Brazilian medical ethics is against its practice as we saw in the analysis of codes of medical ethics.

The New Brazilian Code of Medical Ethics

The most recent Brazilian Code of Medical Ethics enforced on April 13, 2010, promotes better end-of-life care by acknowledging the inevitability of death and encouraging doctors to promote palliative care and good death. We have witnessed some interesting changes, among others: Chapter I, about fundamental principles, admits the "finitude of human life". If one examines the 19 fundamental principles of the previous code of medical ethics (1988), the patient never dies! It is strange, as in the principle, the reality of human death is denied, that it furtively introduces itself in clinical practice (Pessini 2010, 2011).

The current Brazilian Code of Medical Ethics, among the fundamental principles (Chapter I), has two provisions which are in relation to the issue of medical futility. Provision VI states: "The doctor will keep absolute respect for the human being and will always act in their benefit. He will never use his knowledge to cause physical or moral suffering, or something that would put in danger the life of the human being, or to omit and cover attempts against their dignity and integrity." Provision XXII reads: "In the irreversible and terminal clinical situations, the doctor should avoid performing unnecessary diagnostic and therapeutic procedures, and will provide the patients under their attention with all appropriate palliative care." Chapter V, which deals with the "relationships with patients and family members", it regulates medical procedures by saying that the doctor is prohibited from "exaggerating the diagnostic or prognostic seriousness, and complicating the therapeutic" (Article 35). The following Article, No. 36, states that the doctor is forbidden to abandon the patient under their care. Paragraph 2 states that "the doctor will not abandon the patient due to a chronic or incurable illness, and will continue to assist them, even if for palliative care".

This same Chapter V, which deals with the relationship "with patients and family members" (Article 41), says no to the practice of euthanasia in the *caput* and no to the practice of medical futility, and yes to palliative care, in the sole paragraph: Article 36. "The doctor is prohibited from abbreviating the patient's life, even upon the patient's request or upon request of his legal representative. Sole paragraph reads as: "in case of incurable and terminal illness the doctor shall offer the available palliative care, without performing useless or obstinate diagnostic and therapeutic actions, always taking into consideration the patient's expressed will or his legal representative's decision, if the patient is unable to express his wishes" (CFM 2010).

The new code of Brazilian medicine ends up incorporating into its text the essence of Resolution 1805 (November 28, 2006) on Life-Sustaining

Treatment, that caused many discussions in Brazilian society. This issue will be our next point of ethical reflection.

LIFE-SUSTAINING TREATMENT: ETHICAL AND JURIDICAL DISCUSSION

Resolution 1805/2006 of the Federal Council of Medicine is an important ethical document in the context of discussing the problem of good medical care at the end of life in Brazil. This issue was linked with the possibility of opening doors to the practice of euthanasia and the Federal Council of Medicine launched a media campaign to influence public opinion and this has created opportunities for public education regarding end-of-life issues. Without doubt, all this context functioned as a preparation for what would come soon, approval of the new Code of Medical Ethics (2010). Resolution 1805 states:

> "Article 1—The doctor is allowed to limit or suspend medical procedures and treatments that prolong the life of the patient in terminal stage of serious and incurable disease, respecting the person's or the legally responsible person's will.
>
> Paragraph 1—The doctor must explain to the patient or to his legal representative the therapeutic modalities which are appropriate for each situation.
>
> Paragraph 2—The decision referred to in the main section must be substantiated and registered in the medical records.
>
> Paragraph 3—The patient or their legal representative has the right to request a second medical opinion.
>
> Article 2—The patient will continue to receive all necessary care to relieve symptoms that lead to suffering, guaranteeing full comfort, physical, mental, social and spiritual assistance, including assuring him the right of discharge from the hospital."

This resolution elaborated by the Federal Council of Medicine provoked an unprecedented reaction in the sphere of medicine itself, as well as in the Brazilian juridical sphere and general public at large. It was wrongly affirmed that the crime of murder would be characterized if the doctor limits or suspends treatments and procedures that are prolonging the life of a patient in the terminal phase of an incurable disease, thus causing this patient's death (Andrade 2011).

On May 9, 2007, the Federal Public Prosecution Office brought a Public Civil Action against the CFM and asked the Federal Justice to revoke Resolution 1805/2006, alleging that the resolution would be opening doors to the performance of euthanasia, and that the latter is characterized as a crime of murder pursuant to the Brazilian Criminal Code. They claimed that the CFM surpassed the limits of its competence and violated constitutional precepts, especially those designed to protect the inalienable right to life.

The Brazilian Penal Code (1940) does not typify either orthothanasia or euthanasia. According to the perpetrator's conduct, it can fit the provisions for murder, assisted suicide, or can even be atypical. Despite this lack of a typical conduct, in Brazil euthanasia is considered a crime. It is placed under Article 121, which deals with murder. The most elementary social rules are defined by law. In fact, within the latter's scope, the minimally ethical is given by criminal law. The Brazilian Criminal Code of 1940 precedes the technological revolution of the second half of the twentieth century and could not expressly forecast hypotheses of such nature. It is the construction promoted by the current law enforcers that will provide the answers, and for this it is essential to resort to other sources than legal formalism alone.

There already have been perspectives ongoing for several years regarding changes in the special part of that Code. The Criminal Code Draft Bill introduces changes in the Special Part of the Code in force, in Article 121, when dealing with murder.

Thus, we would have, in paragraph 3: "If the crime perpetrator is spouse, companion, ascendant, descendant, brethren, or a person linked to the victim by close ties of affection, and acted due to compassion, upon the latter's request, imputable, and over eighteen years of age, to abbreviate their unbearable physical suffering due to serious and terminal disease, duly diagnosed: Penalty — Confinement, from two to five years."

Paragraph 4 would read as follows: "It does not constitute a crime to fail to maintain somebody's life by artificial means, if death is previously attested by two doctors as imminent and unavoidable, and if there is consent by the patient or, if not conscious, by their spouse, companion, ascendant, descendant, or brethren." Thus we would have the regulation of euthanasia and orthothanasia, respectively, weakening the former and making it clear in the text of the law the nonexistence of an anti-juridical act upon orthothanasia performance. Orthothanasia, from the criminal viewpoint, constitutes an impossible crime, as there is not any crime against life when the life is extinguished by itself. In fact, the vital cycle's natural closing is a common biological fact to the entire mankind, and nobody can escape it.

The Federal Justice accepted the advance decision request contained in the referred public civil action, and preliminarily suspended the validity of CFM Resolution 1805/2006 in 2007. However, after the commission heard about the life termination and CFM program in palliative care, they stopped the case processing, because the Federal Public Prosecution Service, the lawsuit plaintiff, recognized the mistake of their filing and requested that their initial claim be deemed inapplicable, admitting that orthothanasia is not a crime of murder and that the CFM has competence to issue Resolution 1805/2006, as it is a resolution about medical ethics.

Upon the ruling issued by Federal Judge Roberto Luís Luchi Demo, Federal Public Prosecutor Luciana Loureiro Oliveira concluded that (1) The Federal Council of Medicine had competence to issue CFM Resolution 1805/2006, which does not deal with criminal law, but instead with medical ethics and the disciplinary consequences in the face of its noncompliance; (2) orthothanasia does not constitute a crime of murder, construing the Criminal Code in the light of the Federal Constitution; (3) CFM Resolution 1805/2006 did not determine significant modifications in the day-to-day work of the doctors who deal with terminal patients, and therefore did not generate the harmful effects alleged in the public civil action complaint.

Thus, today, CFM Resolution 1805/2006 is fully enforced, and its main concern is with the performance of orthothanasia and wanting to avoid dysthanasia, without having anything to do with the performance of euthanasia, as it was initially feared and judged. Therefore, this resolution is considered constitutional, does not infringe any legal provision, does not represent an apology for murder, nor provides incentives for the perpetration of any criminal or illicit conduct against human life, and is in compliance with the Brazilian legal system.

Cultural and Professional Resistance to Accepting the Concept of Brain Death

In Brazil, the cultural and professional resistance to accepting the concept of brain death promotes the practice of medical futility (dysthanasia). Brain death is equivalent to clinical death, and therefore from the ethical and legal perspective, after it is diagnosed, it is the doctor's obligation to remove life support. The withdrawal of life-sustaining treatment in this situation is not considered euthanasia or any other type of offense against life, as we are facing a situation of a dead and non-terminal patient (Zafalon and Porto 2010, p. 261).

However, if in a brain-dead patient the organs are viable for transplantation the organs will be removed and life support will be turned off without any problem. The point is that if the organs are not viable life support is not turned off, since it is claimed that it would be a euthanasia situation. The brain-dead patient ends up being unnecessarily kept on life support for the maintenance of their vital organs. This clearly is a practice of medical futility or dysthanasia, which wastes medical resources and provokes more suffering to the patient, family members, and health professionals. The question is whether the patient is dead or not. We have situations of much perplexity connected to the family members of the deceased loved one, for instance when they notice that the body is still warm and has a heartbeat, which contrast with algidity (coldness) and the absence of a heartbeat, classic signs of human death.

In the presentation of Resolution 1826/2007, Councilor Gerson Zafalon Martins justifies the complexity of the issue:

"… the CFM recognizes that society is not duly familiarized with this topic, which generates anxiety, doubts and fears, however, if people face this situation in an understanding, humane, and solidary environment. Due to those reasons, this resolution issuance has been justified and allow the ethical, moral and legal discussion of the withdrawal of unnecessary and burdensome treatments, facing death as a complement of life and not as an enemy to be defeated at any cost" (Zafalon and Porto 2010, p. 262).

The CFM developed Resolution 1826/2007 (published in the *Federal Official Journal* on December 6, 2007, in Section I, p. 133) which "provides about the legality and ethical character of the therapeutic procedures and supports suspension upon the brain death determination of a non-donor individual".

Article 1 reads as follows: "It is legal and ethical to withdraw the therapeutic support procedures upon the brain death determination of a non-donor of organs, tissues and human body parts for transplantation purposes, pursuant to the provisions of CFM Resolution No. 1480, of August 21, 1997, and pursuant to Act No. 9434, of February 4, 1997." However, paragraph 1 states: "The fulfillment of the decision mentioned in the caput must be preceded by communication and clarification of brain death to the patient's family members or its legal representative and registered in the medical records."

The case of brain death shows the evolution of cultural attitudes through more information and ethical education. The recognition that in medicine sometimes we face a limit and that trying to cross it, i.e. providing futile medicine (dysthanasia), just causes more suffering for the patient and family members is a positive sign of evolution.

The Role of Advance Directives

The advance directive was started in the USA in 1976, in the prospective autonomy period, which grants decision-making autonomy to patients who had previously registered their living wills. In its beginnings, the American legislation recognized the patients' right to refuse treatments for incurable diseases, the treatment of which would only prolong the painful process of dying, that is, to avoid futile and useless treatment or dysthanasia. It does not have anything to do with possible practices of abbreviation of lives (euthanasia), and instead is a procedure that aims to avoid futile treatment, the prolongation of the painful process of dying.

In Brazil, the discussion about living wills and advance directives is still in the initial stage. The Federal Council of Medicine held in 2010 in São Paulo an interesting workshop to approach this issue, and the Technical Chamber on End of Life and Palliative Care of the Council began an educational initiative for the public as well as medical professionals. We still are at a moment of sensitization and awareness in relation to the importance of this ethical instrument seeking to ensure human dignity, a moment very vulnerable to undue manipulations of and interferences with people's values (Siqueira and Brum 2010).

Far from being another step of bureaucratization of the medical–patient and family relationship, in the more and more plural context in which people find themselves as moral strangers, the advance directive has become an instrument of defense of human dignity. Therefore, it is important that we know, as very accurately defined by Spanish bioethicist Miguel A. Sánchez González, that "the advance directive must primarily serve for the patients to become aware of their treatment alternatives, to get involved in certain choices and to control both the medical assistance provided to them, and the way as their death will occur, everything according to their own life values and objectives" (Sánchez González 2005).

In Brazil, through the Federal Council of Medicine, the discussion about the implementation of living wills and advance directives has started. Let us see what this document consists of. In times of techno-scientific evolution in the sphere of life and health sciences, the technological imperative appeared. This intervention imperative has been overcome little by little, with growing ethical awareness of limits in terms of therapeutic investments, maintaining the functions of vital organs, and end-of-life treatment. The patient's autonomy and the respect for his values, mainly his autonomy in the decision-making process, is getting more popularity and currently nothing happens in terms of treatment decision making without his active participation (Siqueira and Brum 2010). In Brazil's healthcare system, in order to preserve the patient's autonomy and values and to overcome the old medical paternalism, the issue of free and informed consent arose, and more recently advance directives, among them living wills, which are valid for the situations in which the person has become mentally incompetent or entered a permanent state of unconsciousness, are getting more attention.

It is important to restrict the use of advance directives only to the situations of terminal illness and irreversible coma. It is a document in which the patient, when still conscious (and mentally competent), formally renounces certain treatments or interventions that would just add more suffering. Another aspect to be observed is that this document can be revoked at any moment by the patient. It happens sometimes that when the patient becomes critically ill, he decides differently than what he had previously planned. The entire process is based on a dialog, a partnership and collaboration seeking respect for the patient's values and options. In order for us to have free and informed legitimate consent, it is required to have (1) necessary elementary information; (2) understanding about the information; (3) freedom for decision making, without coercion, according to the patient's values; and (4) full capability and consciousness to decide in relation to the issue.

It is important to note that one should be very cautious with forms with microscopic text, signed in a hurry, without the necessary time to clarify any possible doubts. Those documents, in their content, must contain the secure intervention consequences, the frequent and serious risks, as well as all information that a common person needs to know in order to make the decision. Let us not forget that truth and freedom are the essence of free and informed consent, and expressions of loyalty and respect towards the patient.

The Do-Not-Resuscitate (DNR) Order in Brazil

In Brazil, most deaths occur in hospitals, more specifically in intensive care units. While the mortality rate is around 3 to 5%, in adult ICUs it ranges from 20 to 30%, there being distinct clinical and therapeutic differences between patients who die in the wards and in ICUs. In general, patients who die in wards are elderly, suffer from chronic-degenerative illnesses, and in many cases receive comfort measures and/or are submitted to revival when cardio-respiratory arrest occurs. The deaths of patients hospitalized in ICUs makes up 30% of all patients. This figure can reach 70% when the do-not-resuscitate order is enforced and respected, because any kind of therapeutic intervention in this precise case would be just useless and futile.

Cardio-respiratory resuscitation maneuvers occur more frequently when the patients have been hospitalized in ICUs for a short time. In those cases, 40% of resuscitation attempts achieve immediate success; in 25% the resuscitation only prolongs the dying process, and in 6% there is survival without any kind of consequences. Prolonging the dying process causes suffering to all persons involved; patients, families as well as healthcare professionals. Therefore this kind of painful situation should be avoided. The recognition of the legality of Resolution 1805/2006 (Federal Council of Medicine) also eliminates any doubts related to the legality of the non-resuscitation order. The ethical concern here is just to avoid any kind of association with the practice of euthanasia, as well as dysthanasia (AMIB 2009). The CFM through the End of Life and Palliative Care Task Force prepared a resolution in 2009 about the DNR order, which still needs the approval of the Assembly. Following is the essence of its content:

Article 1 reads: "In the cases of incurable and terminal illness, the doctor must provide the patient with all appropriate palliative care, without per-forming useless or obstinate diagnostic and/or therapeutic actions, among them, cardio respiratory resuscitation."

Article 2 reads: "The doctor must register on the medical records, the order of not to resuscitate, collecting the patient's written consent with the respective signature. Such consent can be freely revoked at any time."

Paragraph 1. The doctor must clarify to the patient the diagnostic and/or therapeutic alternatives available for his case. Clarification when a treat-ment is deemed "useless" is necessary. Special attention should be in place if the direct communication may cause immediate harm to the patient or aggravate the patient's clinical conditions even further.

Paragraph 2. The patient is entitled to the constitution of a medical board or to obtain a second opinion about his clinical conditions and about the diagnostic and/or therapeutic alternatives available, before deciding about the DNR order.

Paragraph 3. If the patient maintains verbal communication but is unable to write or sign, the registration of their consent will be made by the doctor, in the presence and with the signature of two witnesses who are independent of the team responsible for the patient's care.

Paragraph 5. The DNR order can be part of the Advance Care Directives, and in this case is part of the medical records of the patient" (CFM 2012).

The great fear in this ethical issue is that when a DNR order is enforced, euthanasia is being performed and the physician becomes vulnerable before the law and can be prosecuted. Therefore, it is still difficult to establish procedures of care at the end of life in Brazil. While Brazilian intensive care physicians usually prefer no-resuscitation approaches, in the Northern Hemisphere removing patients from mechanical ventilation is part of routine care (Santos and Bassitt 2011).

Intensive Care Units and Palliative Care

Although intensive care units are intended to manage potentially recoverable clinically unstable patients, many ICU patients eventually die from multiple organ failure. In addition, some patients with chronic-degenerative diseases are admitted to ICUs due to their underlying diseases. This raises ethical issues related to both the appropriate care of terminal critically ill patients and resource allocation policies (Piva *et al.* 2011). Promotion of better communication and ICU palliative care knowledge may prevent conflicts and improve therapy for critically ill patients. Respect for the patients' and families' socio-cultural and religious values, evaluation of the ethical and practical consequences of the refusal or withdrawal of futile treatments, and the administration of sedation are advised to reduce the suffering of all parties. Proceeding with the Technical Council on End of Life and Palliative Care of the Brazilian Association of Intensive Medicine, considering the previously established concepts and the need for the palliative care of all critically ill patients, the Second Forum of the End of Life Study Group of the Southern Cone of America was conducted in Brasilia in 2010. It aimed to develop recommendations for palliative care for critically ill patients. Following are the recommendations developed by this Forum:

1. Palliative care should be provided to every patient admitted to an intensive care unit (ICU).
2. Intensive care phases should be clarified:

    Phase I. A condition for which the team anticipates better outcomes (recovery versus death or irreversibility). It is judged, respecting beneficence and autonomy, that priority should be given to cure/recovery-focused measures. Palliative care will be provided to relieve the discomfort caused by the illness and the intensive therapy (death unlikely to happen).

Phase II. A condition for which the team perceives a lack of or an insufficient response to the interventions with a growing trend to a fatal outcome or irreversibility. A consensus is established among the team, patient and family member, and priority is given to the best possible quality of life; disease-modifying interventions can be provided when considered by the team and the patient/family to be proportional (death anticipated within days, weeks or months).

Phase III. A condition for which the team acknowledges the disease irreversibility and imminent death, accepting the fatal outcome. Palliative care should be the exclusive type of care provided, and all measures are aimed to improve the quality of life and the patient's/family members' comfort (death anticipated within hours or days).

3. In all phases, customized care should be provided, sufficient to ensure physical, psychological/emotional, and socio-cultural care for the patient and their family, respecting bioethical, deontological and legal perspectives.

4. In all phases, previous guidelines should be verified, as well as interdisciplinary diagnosis, prognosis and therapy evaluations, family members' understanding and the identification of potential conflicts.

5. During the first phase, the care emphasis is placed on the support of the patient's vital systems and on full recovery, but the psychological/emotional comfort of the patient/family should never be neglected.

6. During the second phase, emphasis is shifted to offering and maintaining a set of measures aimed to ensure the physical and psychological/emotional comfort of the patient/family.

7. During the third phase, the emphasis is focused on offering physical and psychological/emotional comfort measures to the patient/family. The importance of the avoidance of starting and/or maintaining unnecessary and futile treatments should be emphasized. Privileging communication and better conditions for the family to stay with the patient and get prepared for the death.

8. During palliative care preferential emphasis should be focused on the patient's welfare, especially regarding preferences and symptom control (pain, discomfort, dyspnea, dry mouth, noisy breathing, etc.).

9. When crossing from the second to the third phase, it is crucial to provide assistance with the decision-making process to the patient and/or
   family to establish a consensus, based on the severity of the condition
   and the patient's/family's preferences and values. The model could be
   either more paternalistic or more participative. The development of
   communications skills is fundamental to providing this assistance
   (Moritz *et al.* 2011, p. 27).

Aiming to improve the care of critically ill patients, the recommendations
focused on the qualifications of the multidisciplinary team that deliver
palliative care. However, there is no need to separate ICU and palliative
care. Palliative care should be included in good ICU practices, both for
adults and for children (Moritz *et al.* 2008).

CONCLUSION

In Brazil, the legal framework for palliative care and end-of-life care is
progressively being revised, as we saw through the reflective ethical jour-
ney in this paper. As in other countries, such regulatory changes are usually complex and progress slowly (Bertachini and Pessini 2011). A recent
study done by Forte *et al.* (2011) presents the results of a questionnaire
submitted to 105 Brazilian ICU physicians selected from 11 ICUs in a
university-affiliated hospital evaluating end-of-life decisions involving a
hypothetical severely brain-damaged patient with no family members or
advance directives. The study has two major findings that goes together
with our convictions in these concluding remarks of the paper: (1) physicians who would not apply do-not-resuscitate orders less frequently
attended end-of-life courses; and (2) almost half of the respondents would
not proceed according to what they believed to be most appropriate for the
patient (i.e. provide less aggressive futile treatment), motivated chiefly by
legal concerns, the fear of being prosecuted. As expected, both the interest
in and reading about end-of-life issues were lower in physicians who
would apply "full code" status than those who would decide to withdraw
life-sustaining therapies.

    Furthermore, it has been demonstrated that younger physicians and ICU
physicians reading at least four articles per year on ethical aspects were

more prone to involve family and nurses in the end-of-life decision-making process, as well as making proactive decisions (Forte *et al.* 2011; Soares and Piva 2012). According to Forte *et al.*, in Brazil, legal and ethical codes remain uncertain, increasing the fear of prosecution for many professionals. Despite these concerns, withdrawal and withholding of life-sustaining treatments are increasingly practiced in Brazil, and in some circumstances, even desired by patients' families. In 2010, the Brazilian Federal Council of Medicine included palliative care as an option during end-of-life care in its Ethical Code and, recently, ethical statements have addressed the possibility of withdrawal of life-sustaining treatment in end-of-life situations. Our study provides evidence that these legal concerns may compel physicians to have a more aggressive attitude during end-of-life care, despite their belief that this approach may not be the best for the patient. This observation raises some concerns about whether Brazil's legal standing on end-of-life issues is protecting patients or causing them harm. This dilemma needs to be addressed in open discussions involving the society in order to improve patient care at the end of life (Forte *et al.* 2011).

This study demonstrates that ethical knowledge positively modifies the end-of-life decision-making process and provides additional evidence that, like any other procedure or intervention performed in ICUs, specific training in end-of-life issues should be formally incorporated into training programs in critical care. So, the key message is that by providing ethics education we can improve the quality of care for patients at the end of their lives.

REFERENCES

Associação de Medicina Intensiva Brasileira (Brazilian Association of Intensive Medicine). 2009. Censo AMIB, São Paulo.

Andrade EO. 2011. A ortotanásia e o Direito Brasileiro. A resolução. 2011. CFM n. 1805/2006 e algumas considerações preliminares à luz do Biodireito Brasileiro. *Revista Bioethikós* 5: 28–34.

Bertachini L and Pessini L. 2011. *Encanto e Responsabilidade no Cuidado da Vida: Lidando com Desafios Éticos em Situações Críticas e de Final de Vida.* São Paulo: Paulinas & Centro Universitário São Camilo.

Brazilian Institute of Geography and Statistics. 2010. Available at: http://www.ibge.gov.br [last visited Dec 20, 2012].

Cassel EJ. 1991. *The Nature of Suffering and the Goals of Medicine.* New York: Oxford University Press.

Conselho Federal De Medicina. Código de Ética Médica resolução CFM n. 1246/88. Diário Oficial da União, 26 de janeiro de 1988, seção 1, pp. 1574–1577.

Conselho Federal De Medicina. 2010. Ortotanásia na Justiça Brasileira. (Documentação). *Revista Bioethikós* 4: 476–486.

Conselho Federal De Medicina. Resolução No. 1931/2009. Ementa: Aprova o Código de Ética Medica. Publicada no D.O.U. de 24 de setembro de 2009, seção I, pp. 90–91.

Forte D, Velasco I, and Park M. 2011. Association between education in EOL, care and variability in EOL practice: A survey of ICU physicians. *Intensive Care Medicine* 38: 404–412.

Fortes P. 2012. SUS, um sistema fundado na solidariedade e na equidade e na equidade e seus desafios. *Vida Pastoral* 52: 22–27.

Martin L. 1996. Saúde e bioética: A arte de acolher e conquistar o bem-estar. *O Mundo da Saúde* 20: 368–373.

Martin L. 1993. *A Ética Médica Diante do Paciente Terminal: Leitura Ético-Teológica da Relação Médico-Paciente Terminal nos Códigos Brasileiros de Ética Médica.* Aparecida: Editora Santuário.

Martin L. 1999. Eutanásia, mistanásia, distanásia, ortotanásia. In: G Cinà, E Locci, C Rocchetta, and L Sandrin, eds. *Dicionário Interdisciplinar da Pastoral da Saúde.* São Paulo: Editora do Centro Universitário São Camilo/ Edições Loyola, pp. 467–482.

Miguel Angel Sánchez González. *A new testament: Vital Testaments and Advance Guidelines*, Faculdade de Ciências Jurídicas do Planalto Central, Year I, Number I, October 2005, Brasília, Federal District, p. 52.

Moritz RD, Deicas A, Rossini JP, Brandão da Silva N, do Lago PM, and Machado FO. 2010. Percepção dos profissionais sobre o tratamento no fim da vida, nas unidades de terapia intensiva da Argentina, Brasil e Uruguai. *Revista Brasileira de Terapia Intensiva* 22: 125–132.

Moritz RD, do Lago PM, de Souza RP *et al.* 2008. End of life and palliative care in intensive care unit. *Revista Brasileira de Terapia Intensiva* 20: 422–428.

Mortiz RD, Deicas A, Capalbo M *et al.* 2011. Second Forum of the "End of Life Study Group of the Southern Cone of America": Palliative care definitions, recommendations and integrated actions for intensive care and pediatric intensive care units. *Revista Brasileira de Terapia Intensiva* 23: 24–29.

Pessini L. 2005. Ethical questions related to end-of-life decisions: The Brazilian reality. In: RJ Blank and JC Merrick, eds. *End-of-Life Decision Making: A Cross-National Study*. Cambridge, MA: MIT Press, pp. 13–31.

Pessini L. 2010. Reflexões bioéticas sobre a distanásia a partir da realidade brasileira. In: DC Ribeiro, ed. *A Relação Médico-Paciente: Velhas Barreiras, Novas Fronteiras*. São Paulo: Centro Universitário São Camilo, pp. 165–195.

Pessini L. 2011. Medicina brasileira e ética: Uma leitura sobre terminalidade e espiritualidade nos códigos de ética médica brasileiros e sobre diretrizes de alguns países. *Revista Vida Pastoral* 52: 28–43.

Pessini L, Paul de Barchifontaine C, and Lolas Stepke F, eds. 2010. *Ibero-American Bioethics: History and Perspectives*. Dordrecht: Springer.

Piva JP, Garcia PCR, and Lago PM. 2011. Dilemmas and difficulties involving end-of-life decisions and palliative care in children. *Revista Brasileira de Terapia Intensiva* 23: 78–86.

Sánchez González MA. 2005. *A New Testament: Vital Testaments and Advance Guidelines*. Faculdade de Ciências Jurídicas do Planalto Central, Year I, Number I, October, Brasília, Federal District, p. 52.

Santos G and Bassitt DP. 2011. End of life in intensive care: Family members' acceptance of orthotanasia. *Revista Brasileira de Terapia Intensiva* 23: 448–454.

Schneiderman LJ. 2008. *Embracing our Mortality: Hard Choices in an Age of Medical Miracles*. Oxford: Oxford University Press.

Siqueira JE and Brum E. 2010. Testamento vital: Conselho Federal de Medicina prepara documento para garantir dignidade na morte. In: DC Ribeiro, ed. *A Relação Médico-Paciente: Velhas Barreiras, Novas Fronteiras*. São Paulo: Centro Universitário São Camilo, pp. 231–255.

Soares M and Piva JP. 2011. Editorial: Physicians just need to be better trained to provide the best care at the end-of-life. *Intensive Care Medicine* 23: 388–390.

Zafalon G and Porto D. 2010. Editorial: Morte encefálica em não doador: quando desligar os aparelhos? *Revista Bioética* 18: 261–262.

CHAPTER THREE

MEDICAL FUTILITY AND END-OF-LIFE ISSUES IN BELGIUM

Jan L Bernheim, Thierry Vansweevelt and Lieven Annemans

SUMMARY

Together with the Netherlands and Luxembourg, Belgium is so far unique in having legalized physician-assisted dying. Because Belgian palliative care is among the most developed in Europe, medically futile treatments at the end of life are likely reduced. Moreover, because -uniquely- Belgian palliative care has largely adopted the possibility of euthanasia, integrating it in "comprehensive palliative care", also the initiation or continuation of palliative care can be avoided by those patients who (have come to) consider it futile. The Belgian model of "comprehensive end-of-life" care is thus able to reduce both medical and palliative futility at the end of life, and likely to do so.

INTRODUCTION AND GENERAL ETHICAL ISSUES

Belgium is no exception among other countries in having to come to grips with medical futility (in Dutch usually called "therapeutische hardnek-kigheid" and in French "acharnement thérapeutique", which best translate as "therapeutic obstinacy"). The motives to discourage or curb medical futility, as elsewhere, are at the same time clinical, ethical and economi-cal. Medical futility occurs either at the initiative of physicians or at the request of patients, and sometimes both, when physicians and patients or their representatives concur in wishing for physiologically futile treatment to be initiated or prolonged. Physiologically futile treatment has no physi-ological benefit because it is ineffective. Examples are prescribing an antibiotic for a benign viral infection or cardiopulmonary resuscitation of a patient with end-stage myocardial dysfunction. Physiological futility is based on objective, evidence-based criteria. It is bad medicine, because it violates all of the four classical medical-ethical values (Beauchamp and Childress 1979): it does no good to the patients, it harms them, it often violates their autonomy and it causes injustice as it drains resources which are denied to others who need them (Niederman & Berger 2010).

Physician-initiated medical futility, when its motives are to serve the interests of the caregiving staff or institution, can be an extreme case of "strong" paternalism, where against the patient's wishes, others decide for patients to do them fictitious good and even to harm them, It can also belong to "weak" paternalism when it is done without the patient having a preference. If the latter situation results from the patient not having been informed of the options and issues at stake, such medical futility is both unethical and illegal.

If, in contrast, medical futility occurs at the explicit request of the informed patient, against the "physiologic" judgment of the physicians who, if they accept, then place the patient's values above their own, we have an ethically quite different situation. This is what has been termed "normative futility" (Younger 1990). The patient's values can then be argued to be served since the patients exert their autonomy and *feel* they benefit from futile treatment. In such cases, only the justice principle is violated. Futile treatment at the request of the patient poses a difficult problem of conflicting interests: the values of the individual patient are then at odds with the doctor's and the interest of society. An intermediary sub-category of medical futility is when it is prompted by the patient's relatives, in the best of cases to soothe their conscience, in the worst for secondary gain. There are for Belgium no epidemiological data on which of physician or patient-prompted futility is -quantitatively, i.e. in terms of number of cases and financial burden- the most important problem.

Another complication relative to straightforward cases is when the values at stake are not binary or categorical (e.g. life prolongation of a permanent vegetative condition or not), but quantitative (e.g. life prolongation for a minimal time or not, or life prolongation at the cost of severe suffering). In the latter cases, there is problem of proportionality and a balance of pros and cons has to be made.

In the USA, although the debate is still ongoing (Schneiderman 2011), much jurisprudence and some jurisdiction seem to have gone beyond the negative right of a patient to refuse treatment to the positive right to obtain treatment, even when physiologically futile. According to some case law, this is also when the demand comes not from the patients themselves, but from relatives (e.g. who attach normative value to the continuation of physical life of the body of an irreversibly unconscious person) (Veatch 2009). Thus, the autonomy of the patient (or their relatives) seems to be given priority over the autonomy of the caregiver, both for refusing any treatment and for demanding physiologically futile treatment (Lantos *et al.* 1989). Concisely put, concerns over medical futility seems in the USA to be more concerned with protecting the physician from patients' futile demands than with protecting the patient from physician-driven futile treatment. Not so in Belgium, where only the negative patient right to refuse treatment is legally enforced, and also –theoretically- the duty of physicians to refrain from futile treatment, as will be detailed below. However, the contrast between the USA and Belgium is likely to become less marked since also in America physician-driven futile treatment is under increased scrutiny (Earle *et al.* 2008, Ho *et al.* 2011).

THE HEALTHCARE SYSTEM IN BELGIUM

Belgium is a constitutional monarchy with a parliamentary system of democracy. Over the last decades it has become an increasingly decentralized federal state, with ever-increasing devolution of competences to the

Flemish and Walloon regions and the (bilingual) Brussels-capital region. Federal Belgium, Flanders, Wallonia and Brussels all have their own parliaments and administrations. Taking a broad view, as more and more judicial, ecological, financial and economic decision-making has gone to the European level, and in Belgium ever more competences are devolved to regional authorities, the responsibilities of the Belgian federal government are gradually shrinking. Only about 60% of government expenditure is federal. Only the ministries of defense, foreign affairs, finances and justice are wholly federal competences, as is to a large extent social security. There is a federal Belgian minister of health and social affairs, but also the regions have such administrations. This devolution has the advantage of reducing the distance between government and the citizenry, but it often entails a complex, arduous and lengthy decision-making process.

Belgium's population, which has been slightly growing over the last decades due to immigration, stands at about 11 million in 2012. Children (0–17 years), adults (18–64 years), and elderly people (≥65 years) constitute 20.6%, 62.4% and 17.1% of the total population, respectively. The average lifespan in Belgium was 77.36 years for men and 82.64 years for women in 2010 (statbel.fgov.be).

Belgium has universal health insurance, which is financed not by taxes but by contributions to social security by individual citizens, including employers, employees and also pensioners. In addition, people increasingly tend to buy complementary private insurance. Medical technological progress, the aging of the population, unemployment at ~9% and a tendency over the last decades to ever shorter working careers (during which time citizens contribute to social security) because of longer education and earlier retirement put the social health-insurance system under increasingly severe financial strain.

The health-care delivery system in Belgium can be characterized as liberal (free choice of caregivers, fee-for-service), with strong cooperative and solidarity corrections. Citizens are members of the non-profit cooperatives called "mutualities" which reimburse them of (the largest part of) their health-care expenditures. In effect, the mutualities are the executive branch of the National Institute for Health and Disability Insurance (NIHDI). People choose one of 7 mutualities, some with a political denomination (Christian, Socialist, Liberal…), others neutral or independent mutualities. All are entrusted by the NIHDI to deliver core services such as (partial) reimbursement of health-care expenses and home nursing care. Mutualities in addition offer various optional services such as preventive care and children's vaccination. Some mutualities also run out-patient clinics.

The NIHDI insurance coverage includes medicines, physician consultations, interventions, lab tests and imaging, hospitalization and nursing care.

In 2010, only 0.96% of residents of Belgium were uninsured (ww.riziv. be), many of them illegal refugees or immigrants. However, their emergency needs are met by municipal "public assistance" and in a few cases charities. Insured members pay a varying % of medical expenses out-of-pocket, ranging from 0% for approved treatments for life-threatening conditions to 100% for e.g. some optional aesthetic surgery, depending on perceived need. Burdens on the elderly, children, and low-income individuals are lower. Medicines are reimbursed between 100% for cost-effective drugs used in life-threatening diseases such as cancer and 0% for drugs which by the NIHDI are judged not effective or not cost-effective.

The medical profession is subject to the oversight of the Ordre des Médecins/Orde van Geneesheren (Medical Disciplinary Board or Medical Order), an elected body with provincial councils, which issues guidelines and adjudicates disputes and complaints. It is also subject to the Provincial Medical Inspection. Most doctors and paramedics are members of unions and scientific and/or professional interest associations. A Federal Health Council advises on quality of care and prevention, but has no jurisdiction over the payment system. Health-care delivery is at three levels: primary (including general practitioners (GP), senior citizens' and care and nursing homes, with a nursing staff but where residents have their own GP), secondary (including municipal and regional hospitals) and tertiary (university hospitals and specialized referral centers). Patients choose their GP, but these are not gatekeepers to the consultation of specialists, who can be consulted directly. This has the advantage of high accessibility, but the drawback of some duplication of e.g. examinations and some overconsumption of services. The overall density of Belgian physicians is about 40,000, of which 25,000 are specialists.

Belgian GP's have a very high density (1.3 active GPs per 1000 inhabitants), practice an exceptionally high rate of home calls (26% of all consultations) (FOD Volksgezondheid 2011) and are on record as usually quite knowledgeable on their patients' psycho-social environment.

The number of hospital beds is 6.7 per 1000 inhabitants. The average duration of hospitalization in 2008 was 5 days, down from 5.9 days in 2005. The average cost of care per year for patients without a chronic disease is €1.381, whereas for chronic patients this amounts to €10.827 (www.riziv.fgov.be). The % of lifelong healthcare expenditure used during the last month of life has not yet been calculated.

As for output results, Belgian health indicators and outcomes are generally considered to be in the upper-middle range of European countries. According to the European Values Study the confidence of Belgians in their health care system rose from 87% in 1999 to 92% in 2008, after Iceland the highest in Europe (European Values Study 2008 and Halman 2011). The 2002 legalization of euthanasia, the generalization of palliative care and the law on patients' rights, probably the most important changes in health care in the past decade, rather seem to have increased the confidence of the public.

Under the auspices of the NIHDI there are yearly negotiations on the organization of care, the registration of "heavy" equipment and services such as NMR and PET-CT and selection for and level of reimbursement of services. Caregivers are represented by their unions and patients by the mutualities. Physicians who adhere to the convention (the vast majority) pledge to apply the national fees for most of their working time and are rewarded by a payment to their personal retirement plan.

Planning, regulation and management of specialized or multidisciplinary care is organized by the NIHDI. Registered regional or university cancer centers must offer multidisciplinary services and tumor-board deliberation of cases. Other examples are officially registered centers for assisted procreation and genetic counseling. The objectives of this system are to ensure optimal distribution of state-of-the art health care and to control expenses. The current politically decided benchmark is a yearly growth of health-care expenditure of 2% (excluding inflation). In the recently shrinking economy, this is a major challenge.

ETHICS IN END OF LIFE SITUATION IN BELGIUM

Epidemiological Data

The mortality rate in Belgium is 0.958% per year, with 105,094 annual deaths. Place of death is a hospital in 52%, the home in 22%, a care and nursing home in 22% and 2% elsewhere. This falls well short of expressed patients' preferences, of which too few physicians are aware (Meeussen *et al.* 2009). In Flanders (Belgium) 72% of the citizens in case of advanced cancer wish to die at home and 10% in a hospice or palliative care unit (Gomes *et al.* 2012). Causes of death are cardiovascular disease (32%), cancer (27.1%), respiratory diseases (11%) and unnatural deaths (accidents, suicide) (6.4%) (www.statbel.be). Palliative care, the treatment modality aimed at "total" physical, emotional, social and spiritual comfort at the end of life, at the exclusion of further attempts to prolong survival by clinically burdensome and costly disease-directed treatment, is explicitly an alternative to medical futility. The penetration of palliative care is high in Belgium: 41% of all non-sudden deaths are preceded by organized multidisciplinary palliative care during the last three months of life (~30% of all deaths), (Van den Block *et al.* 2008). Roughly on a par with the Netherlands and the United Kingdom, Belgium belongs to a cluster of European countries with the highest level of development of palliative care (Chambaere *et al.* 2011). The Benelux countries, are currently the only worldwide to have legalized and regulated euthanasia (Belgium and the Netherlands in 2002 and Luxembourg in 2009). Life-ending acts at the explicit request of the patient are legal (under strictly defined conditions[1]) when the patient considers the initiation or pursuit of palliative care futile.

Contrary to official stances elsewhere (Materstvedt *et al.* 2003), in Belgium palliative care and euthanasia are not at all opposed propositions,

---

[1]Euthanasia is legally defined as intentionally terminating the life of another person, at this person's request. It is legal under 2002 Belgian Law under the following conditions:

- Repeated consistent request, under no external pressure, in writing (with witnessed written advance directives for the future case of irreversible incompetence).
- Competent adult patient
- "Intolerable" and irreversible suffering, physical and/or mental
- Caused by an irreversible medical condition
- Patient duly informed of alternatives, including palliative care

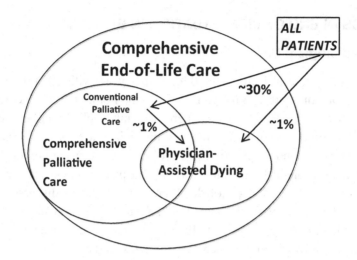

Fig. 1.   The Belgian model of comprehensive end-of-life care.

but were historically synergistic. The first palliative care initiatives were taken by advocates of legal euthanasia, who went on to prominently contribute to the development of the palliative care system. Vice-versa, adequate palliative care made the legalization of euthanasia ethically and politically acceptable. The Belgian model (Figure 1) is best described as "Comprehensive End-of-Life Care" (Bernheim *et al.* 2008).

The Venn diagram shows that comprehensive Palliative care is conventional palliative care (as practiced in countries without legal euthanasia) offering also the option of euthanasia. A reasonable estimate based on the study of Belgian patients during the last three months of their lives is that about 30% of all deaths (41% of all non-sudden deaths) are preceded by organized multidisciplinary palliative care, and that about 2% die with euthanasia, half of them after a palliative care pathway (Van den Block

- Carried out by physician, after consultation of nursing team and a competent colleague, who must examine the patient, verify the fulfillment of the legal requirements and write his findings in the patient file
- The physician must be present till the death of the patient
- If the patient is not expected to die within the foreseeable future, two colleagues must be consulted and a moratorium of one month respected
- Report to the Federal Control & Evaluation Commission of Euthanasia for accountability. Auditing in cases of doubt. Referral to the public prosecutor possible.

et al. 2008). Significant numbers of caregivers are conscientious objectors to euthanasia, which is respected by the law and in practice. The physician refusing to carry out euthanasia must in due time inform his patient of this, giving also the reasons for his refusal (Art. 14 of the Euthanasia Law). If the refusal is on medical grounds, this must be documented in the patient's file. The evolution of the epidemiology of end of life decision with a possible or certain life-abbreviating effect is shown in Table 1.

Table 1.   Frequency of Medical End-of-Life Practices in Flanders, Belgium, 1998, 2001 and 2007.*

Variables	1998	2001	2007
Total annual death, No.	56,354	55,793	54,881
Death in study sample, No.	3,999	5,005	6,202
Response rate %	48.2	58.9	58.4
Deaths included in analyses, No.	1,925	2,950	3,623
Sudden deaths % (95% CI)	33.3 (31.2–35.5)	34.1 (32.2–36.1)	31.9 (30.0–33.8)
Medical end-of-life practices that certainly or possibly hastened death % (95% BI)	39.3 (37.0–41.6)	38.4 (36.6–40.3)	47.8 (45.9–49.8)
Use of life-ending drug	4.4 (3.5–5.5)	1.8 (1.4–2.4)	3.8 (3.2–4.5)
With patient's explicit request (Euthanasia)	1.1 (0.7–1.7)	0.3 (0.2–0.5)	1.9 (1.6–2.3)
Physician-assisted suicide	0.12 (0.04–0.36)	0.01 (0–0.1)	0.07 (0.02–0.2)
Ending life without patient's explicit request	3.2 (2.4–4.1)	1.5 (1.1–2.0)	1.8 (1.3–2.4)
Intensified alleviation of pain symptoms	18.4 (16.6–20.4)	22.0 (20.5–23.6)	26.7 (25.1–28.4)
Withholding or withdrawing life-prolonging treatment	16.4 (14.7–18.3)	14.6 (13.2–16.1)	17.4 (15.9–19.0)
Continues deep sedation % (95% BI)	NA	8.2 (7.2–9.4)	14.5 (13.1–15.9)

*All percentages were adjusted for stratification (according to the underlying cause of death as indicated on the death certificate and the estimated corresponding likelihood of an end-of-life decision having been made) and for characteristics of deaths (age and sex of the patient and place and cause of death). CI denotes confidence interval and NA not available.

The total number of medical end-of-life decisions with a possible or certain life shortening effect increased from 39,3% in 1998 to almost half of all deaths (47.8%) in 2008 (Bilsen *et al.* 2009, Chambaere *et al.* 2010b). The increase was almost entirely attributable to intensified treatment of pain and symptoms with a possible life-abbreviating effect. There was no evidence of vulnerable patients being more at risk of euthanasia. On the contrary, e.g. persons over 80 years old were and remained under-represented among euthanasia recipients (Rietjens *et al.* 2012). Continuous deep sedation is an ever increasingly applied modality of end of life care. Palliative sedation is the keeping comatose of (pre-) terminal patients until their death, whether or not with "windows" of consciousness (in which case it is called "controlled sedation"), with or without continued administration of fluid and nutrition. The latter form of end of life is sometimes considered as "slow euthanasia", and is quite common in palliative care.

The evolutions between 1998 and 2007 reflect the ever growing impact of palliative care because what most increased are the practices belonging to the standard armamentarium of conventional palliative care. The year of 2001, with a lower number of medicinal life terminations, is a particular case because this is when the euthanasia law was being debated and there were more indictments, resulting in more legal insecurity. The incidence of euthanasia rose from 1.1% in 1998 to 1.9% in 2008. In 2008 euthanasia was practiced more in the patient's home (50.3%), and more in cancer (80.2%), with younger patients (only 20.4% of euthanasia cases were in patients older than 80). The administering of drugs with the explicit intention to shorten survival without the patient's explicit request decreased from 3.2% to 1.8% (Van den Block *et al.* 2009). Presumably, most of these cases are now euthanasia. They are vehemently objected to by opponents of euthanasia (Pereira 2011) whose arguments are criticised (Downie *et al.* 2012). These unrequested life terminations were specifically studied in 2007. They were compared to euthanasia cases (by definition upon explicit request) and to all deaths. The drugs administered were usually not barbiturates and muscle relaxants, as for euthanasia, but opiates, whose lethal effect is improbable. In contrast to euthanasia a majority of patients are here older than 80 years (52.7%), unrequested life termination occurs in two-thirds of cases in a hospital, and two-thirds with diseases other than cancer, namely less chronic diseases, with a less predictable course, offering less opportunity for advance planning. The vast majority were agonal patients who had become incompetent, 70% of them comatose and 21% demented. In eighty per cent, the decision was deliberated with family. Whereas in euthanasia, family also expressed the wish for life termination in only 25% of the cases, this was fifty per cent for unrequested life abbreviation. In half of cases the estimated life abbreviation was less than 24 hours (whilst in euthanasia it was so short in only 11.4%). The category of "administering of drugs with the explicit intention to shorten survival without the patient's explicit request" in the death-certificate epidemiological studies in fact results from two questions only on "life-abbreviating intention" and "explicit request", respectively. Euthanasia and unrequested life abbreviation are clinically quite different practices, largely in other patients and circumstances and the latter must be understood as compassionate intended abbreviation of the agonal phase of dying. According to most physicians in most countries, this belongs to traditional humane medical practice, but it is revealed only in those few countries in which epidemiological studies of the end of life have been carried out and in which physicians are less prone to applying the "double effect principle" (McIntyre 2004, White et al. 2011). This said, the statistical data do not exclude clandestine unethical practices, but if such occur, they are rare, and because of increased scrutiny and societal control, probably less likely than in the past.

Between 1998 and 2007 medical end-of-life decisions were increasingly discussed with patients, their family, colleagues and nursing staff, which suggests more carefulness. It should be noted that in 1998, 44% of end-of-life decisions were discussed with nursing staff with a peak of 66% in 2001 and a decrease to 51% in 2007, which leaves to be desired (the peak in 2001 may reflect the then prevailing legal insecurity and a few indictments of doctors by e.g. nurses or family who objected to euthanasia and/or had other grievances).

Some other numbers are still less than fully satisfactory. In 2007, in about 20% of drug-mediated life abbreviations, no colleague was consulted and the reporting rate of euthanasia, though gradually increasing towards 80%, was still suboptimal. The latter can be inferred from the difference between the number of cases reported to the Federal Control and Evaluation Commission (Smets et al. 2010) and the estimates of euthanasia incidence in the successive population-based epidemiological studies (Bilsen et al. 2009, Chambaere et al. 2010a, Van den Block et al. 2009).

In sum, during the preparation of the legalisation of euthanasia Belgian doctors increasingly applied the precepts of conventional palliative care avoiding futile disease-directed treatments and since legalisation even more so. The recent epidemiological data on end of life practices confirm the concomitance of palliative care and euthanasia. In hospital-based palliative care units, prior to non-sudden deaths, more possibly or certainly life abbreviating end of life decisions are made than in general wards. For euthanasia this is 3% versus 1%. These data were obtained with a different methodology from the preceding death certificate studies (Van den Block *et al.* 2007), via the Sentinel Network of General Practitioners (GPs), a surveillance panel of GPs who are representative for all GPs and nursing home physicians in Belgium. For these studies the sentinel GPs described the pathway of their patients who died in 2005–2006. The relationship was investigated between (possibly) life-abbreviating end-of-life decisions and having received multidisciplinary specialised palliative care during the last three months of life. When palliative care had been used, euthanasia was not less frequent (there was a statistically non-significant excess of euthanasia in palliative care), and significantly more end of life decisions with an explicitly life-abbreviating objective were made (odds ratio 1.5, 95% CI 1.1 tot 2.1), (Van den Block *et al.* 2007, Chambaere *et al.* 2010b). All these differences between palliative care and standard care can, to a certain extent, be due to factors of patient selection such as a heavier symptom burden in palliative care patients, but they prove at any rate that in Belgium there is no contradiction between palliative care and life-abbreviating practices. Palliative care in Belgium thus not only replaces futile medical treatment, but also accepts that some patients consider further palliative care as futile.

An attempt at calculation of the aggregate economic benefits of the taking of life-abbreviating end-of-life decisions (ELD) was based on the death-certificate-based epidemiological study of 1998 (Deliens *et al.* 2000), in which the physicians (anonymously) describing the cases also estimated the amount of time irreversibly suffering survival was abbreviated by the end of life decision. Survival after all types of life-abbreviating end of life decision in Flanders was reduced by a total of 126,000 patient-days, on average seven days per patient (Bernheim 2002). Gielen *et al.* (2010) reported a cost of €14,228 for the last 6 months of life. The cost in the last month was €6,298 for cancer patients and €4,311 for non cancer patients. Assuming a distribution of patients as in Chambaere *et al.* (2010b), with 65% of end of life decisions made in cancer patients, the average cost in the last month is estimated at €5,599. Hence, the impact of a reduction in life span of 7 days on the health care budget could be conservatively (assuming a constant cost in the last month) estimated at €1,306 per patient. Since in about half of all ~100,000 deaths annual deaths in Belgium an end of life decision supposedly avoiding futile treatment is made, the annual savings on the basis of the 1998 epidemiological data can be roughly estimated as €65,000,000.

MEDICAL FUTILITY: LEGAL, PROFESSIONAL RULES AND GUIDELINES

Every hospital or district by law has its pluralistically composed ethical committee dealing with specific problems. For general bioethical issues, there is the Federal Advisory Committee for Bioethics, which is composed of ethicists, lawyers and representatives of the organized religious and philosophical constituencies, including secular humanism. Its report to Parliament in 1998 was pivotal in bringing about the euthanasia legislation.

There is no specific legislation dedicated to medical futility in Belgium. However, indirectly the legislation concerning the mandatory insurance on health care and benefits is pertinent Article 73, §1 of this law determines that in principle physicians have therapeutic freedom, but they must refrain from futile or unnecessary expensive treatments supported by the health insurance (www.riziv.fgov.be).

In the Medical Order's professional code of conduct a few articles refer to medical futility (without using the term). For instance, Article 36 and 49 Code Medical Conduct states; 'a physician must avoid and may refuse treatments which have no sufficient medical indication'. Also, in the context of the end of life of the patient, Article 97 of the same Code says that the physician must prevent therapeutic obstinacy.

Further, several Belgium institutions are competent to issue guidelines: the Federal Control and Evaluation Commission on Euthanasia, the Federal Advisory Committee on Bioethics, The Royal Academy of

Medicine, etc. None of the advisory bodies have elaborated specific ethical guidelines on medical futility. Nonetheless there is an advice recommendation on "do not resuscitate" (DNR) orders from the Federal Advisory Committee on Bioethics which indirectly deals with this topic.

Besides these federal advisory bodies, each hospital is obliged to have a committee on medical ethics (The Law Concerning Hospitals 2008). These committees advise on medical experimentation and on the ethical aspects of hospital care, including medical futility. It is always possible that a local committee on medical ethics establishes some ethical rules on medical futility. The ethical rules issued by a local ethical committee or from a federal advisory body are guidelines and are never legally binding.

In principle physicians have a legally protected therapeutic freedom or professional autonomy: they decide which means must be used to make a diagnosis and treat the patient (The Law Concerning Healthcare Professions 1967). This freedom entails also the right to accept or to refuse the treatment of a patient. An exception to this freedom is when a patient needs urgent treatment (Article 422, Penal Code). Further, a physician can discontinue treating his patient, e.g. when the physician and the patient do not trust each other anymore, on condition that the physician assures the continuity of care by another physician (Art. 8 of the Law of 1967). Not every act by a physician is a medical act. In order to be recognized as a medical act and therefore protected by legislation, the act must be carried out by a physician and preceded by the informed consent of the patient or his legal representative. However, the act must have a preventive, diagnostic or therapeutic goal, including palliative care (Art. 2 of the Law of 1967 and Art. 2 of the Law on Patient's Rights of 2002). Hence, strictly speaking, a physician who performs a futile treatment is not protected by the legislation concerning the execution of medical acts, and could be prosecuted for assault and battery (Art. 418, Penal Code). Given the legal fact that a physician must abstain from futile treatment, it is important to know what is meant by futile treatment. First, it must be emphasized that medical futility is not limited to the end-of life context. In other circumstances physicians may prescribe an examination, a treatment or a drug, e.g. to reassure the patient or because the patient wants this, without any medical indication. Prescribing an antibiotic for a benign common viral illness, for instance, will not have any effect and is futile (Baily 2011). However, without any doubt, the most complex situation arises at the end of life when conflicts between physician and the patient or his family concern matters of life and death.

In accordance with American views (Obade 2011), Belgian legal authors (Delbeke 2012 and Lemmens 2012) recently distinguished four types of medical futility. First is Physiologic futility, when a treatment is futile because it has no physiological benefit and is therefore ineffective and useless. Prescribing an antibiotic for a viral illness or cardiopulmonary resuscitation of a patient with end-stage myocardial dysfunction are cases in point. This type of futility is based on objective evidence.

The second is Quantitative futility: the treatment has some potential effect, but the probability of success is so low that the treatment is considered not to be reasonable. An example is the reanimation of old patients with a severe irreversible chronic disease when the chance of success is less than 5% (Delbeke 2012).

The third group is Economic futility: a treatment is futile when there is some potential effect, but the treatment is considered too costly with regard to the magnitude of this effect (Obade 2011). The goal of this approach is cost control and justice in the allocation of resources.

Finally, the fourth is Qualitative futility: a treatment is futile when the result which it can achieve is not sufficient (Leenen *et al.* 2007). Qualitative futility is also described as disproportional futility. A treatment is futile when there is no reasonable improvement of the state of health of the patient or there is a disproportion between the means of the treatment and the (poor) result of the treatment (Federal Advisory Committee on Bioethics 2007). Disproportional futility comes close to economic futility.

The overarching principle for these considerations is the obligation to always do a cost-benefit analysis, where costs can be both economical and clinical (e.g. side effects and other adverse consequences of treatment), and benefits can be physiological, psychological or social. Cost-benefit analysis can be considered as belonging to the obligatory means of clinical practice.

Sadly, for the end of life, unlike in e.g. Spain (Gómez-Batiste *et al.* 2006, Paz-Ruiz *et al.* 2009), such studies are still lacking in Belgium.

MEDICAL FUTILITY: WHO DECIDES?

The question who decides arises in all four types of medical futility. The ideal scenario which can also be found in the Law on Patient's Rights is of course the principle of *shared decision making* (Mitchell *et al.* 1993, Delbeke 2012). According to Article 7 of the Patient's Right Law, the physician has a duty to inform the patient about the relevant aspects of his illness and the treatment. In current situation, physicians inform the patients (or their legal representatives) about their illness and suggest a particular treatment or no treatment. Together they can choose one of the options which both can fully support. When physician and patient disagree about starting or continuing a treatment, the physician has the duty to explain his medical arguments and try to convince the patient. If the disagreement remains, someone will have to decide. A distinction must be made depending on whether it is the patient or the physician who refuses the treatment at the end of life. The Law on Patients' Rights (Article 8), determines that the patient has the absolute right to refuse a treatment. The physician has the duty to respect the will of the patient not to be treated, even if this hastens his death. Hence, when the informed patient refuses a treatment, even life prolonging, at the end of his life, physicians must respect this wish.

Alternatively, it is the physician who refuses to administer a (futile) treatment. In principle, it is the physician who is considered to be the most suitable agent to decide about futility on the basis of medical criteria. Taking this into account, *physiologic futility* does not seem to cause many legal or ethical problems. There is a broad consensus that a physician has no obligation to perform a physiologically futile treatment (Nys 2005, Tack and Balthazar 2007, and Federal Advisory Committee on Bioethics 2007). Even when a patient asks his physician to perform such a treatment, the physician has the right, and strictly speaking even the obligation, to refuse a physiologically futile treatment. The physician has the obligation to inform the patient about the reasons for this refusal. Hence, it is the physician who decides about performing or not performing such type of futile treatment. If the patient still wants it, he can always decide to choose another physician. Normally, this other physician should also refuse the ineffective treatment.

The other types of futility raise more legal problems because they entail a more subjective value judgment. In that case the decision should be a joint one by physician and patient. But what happens in case of disagreement? According to the majority of the Belgian legal doctrine, in case of quantitative of qualitative futility the physician can never be forced to give a treatment which he deems futile (Genicot 2010, Vansweevelt 2003). In the only publicized judicial verdict on futility in Belgium, the court decided that a physician has the right to abstain from reanimation of a dehydrated, senile and mute patient with respiratory problems in the terminal stage of Pick disease. Reanimation would only have maintained the patient in a vegetative state. The court decided that the physician acted humanely and did the right thing by deciding not to reanimate this patient (Court Case 1991).

Also the Medical Order advises that a physician should stop or withhold a treatment when on medical grounds it is clear that there is no hope for a *reasonable* improvement and life prolonging treatments will not increase the comfort of the patient (Medical Order Advice 2003). According to the Bioethics Federal Advisory Committee a physician can never be coerced to start or continue a useless or futile treatment, which includes quantitative and qualitative futility (Advice No. 41, on DNR code, 2007). The only duty of the physician is to arrange for the continuity of care by another physician.

However, some authors have recently disagreed with the mainstream view. They defend the view that the patient should make the definitive decision about a futile treatment because of the patient's autonomy and because the patient is the best qualified to judge what is an acceptable quality of life (Delbeke 2012, Lemmens 2012).

Because it is difficult for the patient to coerce a physician to carry out a treatment, some hospitals have established internal procedures to resolve this kind of disputes. Most of the times, the hospital ethics committee provides an ethical advice about the futile nature of the proposed treatment. But this problem-resolution mechanism can be criticized because the ethics committee is not an independent institution, but is composed in majority of members of the hospital staff, who can be influenced by financial and professional considerations. In case of continuing disagreement between physician and patient, ultimately the court can be addressed.

However, most courts, commentators and physicians agree that the court-room is not the appropriate venue to settle such disputes (Bassel 2010). Some (American) courts refused to settle futility disputes and stated to lack the necessary expertise to make a decision about terminating or continuing life support (Betancourt vs Trinitas Hospital 2009).

In Belgium, it appears that such disagreements between physicians and their patients or their representatives are quite rare. There is almost no jurisprudence in Belgium concerning end of life and futility disputes.

HOW ARE DECISIONS MADE IN CASES OF FUTILE CARE AND WHO MAKES THEM?

Most Belgians professionals probably agree that the general principle of "shared decision making" is to be followed (Löfmark & Nilstun 2002). In the past, a generally rather paternalistic stance was recommended by the Medical Disciplinary Board. For example, fatal diagnoses were as a rule not to be communicated to patients, and if they were, only 'with due precautions'. The broad principles of "full" information, informed consent and joint decision making are now endorsed by both the health-care professions and the general public. However, the practical implementation of these lofty ideals is complicated. Empirical research has shown that among patients there is a broad spectrum of preferences for the level of information, ranging from "none at all" to "all" (Deschepper et al. 2008). Also patient preferences for the degree of their own and their families' involvement in decision making vary widely (Pardon et al. 2009, Pardon et al. 2010). Moreover, these preferences change over time as the patient's situation evolves (Pardon et al. 2012a). Patient preferences are often not met (Pardon et al. 2011, Pardon et al. 2012b). These findings support the principle of individually tailored physician-patient interactions, along the lines of "Patient-physician Information and Communication Covenants" (ICC), as proposed several years ago (Bernheim 2001). The ICC procedure aims to let the patient choose within the whole range of physician-patient interactions, including the paternal-filial type. However, covenants are always re-negotiable. It should be noted that, *parental* is to be distinguished from paternalistic. In the former case it is the patient who takes the initiative to assume a filial position and who asks the doctor to be parental. This situation realises what is called "weak" paternalism. A doctor-patient relationship is (strongly) *paternalistic* when it is the physician who takes the initiative to assume such a position. In principle the agenda of an ICC must include a list of items as proposed by Winkler *et al.* (2011).

Qualitative research suggests that oncologists may be under no illusion as to the response rate of aggressive treatments in advanced cancer, but feel that they cannot deny patients hope that may be futile. The authors conclude: "the trend to greater use of chemotherapy at the end of life could be explained by patients' and physicians' mutually reinforcing attitudes of "not giving up" and by physicians' broad interpretation of patients' quality of life, in which taking away patients' hope by withholding treatment is considered harmful" (Buiting *et al.* 2011). Advance systematic end-of-life discussions between patient and physician in advanced cancer patients have been shown to reduce aggressive and therefore often futile treatment during the last phase of life (Mack *et al.* 2012). Also, early supportive involvement of palliative care was proven to improve not only quality of life, but even survival duration, thus *ex absurdo* proving that some pre-terminal aggressive cancer treatment is futile (Earle *et al.* 2008).

THE LINK BETWEEN MEDICAL FUTILITY AND EUTHANASIA IN BELGIUM

The issues of patient rights, palliative care and euthanasia have been and still are strongly linked in the Belgian polity. This is made clear by the fact that the three laws on patient rights, palliative care and euthanasia were enacted together as a package by the federal Parliament in the spring of 2002. These laws are probably the most important changes in health care in Belgium in the last few decades. In the Belgian model of comprehensive end-of-life care, in conformity with the patients' rights law, the decision of what is futile is primarily the patient's (or in case of incompetence their parents or designated persons of confidence). This is implemented even when a competent adult refuses a life-saving act for e.g. religious reasons, as in the case of Jehovah's witnesses (who however cannot exercise the right of refusal of treatment for their child). However, no physician is compelled to carry out a medically futile act. The same principles apply in end of life situations: a patient may consider life-prolonging treatments as futile, as they can also consider the initiation or continuation of palliative care as futile, and request euthanasia. Here again, no physician is under any obligation to carry out euthanasia. If they are conscientious objectors, they are morally and deontologically (as enforced by the Belgian Medical Order) expected to refer the patient to a permissive colleague. However, this obligation has not yet been legally imposed.

CONCLUSION

Together with the Netherlands, Belgium has a strong record of research in palliative care and end-of-life issues (Chambaere *et al.* 2011). Arguably, taking all bioethical legislations together, it is the most liberal country: it is a net exporter of organs for transplantation thanks to its "opting out" law on organ procurement, its legislation on abortion and on assisted procreation and reproductive experimentation is very permissive, same-sex marriage is legal, its development of palliative care is among the highest, and it has legalized euthanasia. Its percentage of people in dialysis treatment for end-stage renal disease is among the highest in the world, illustrating an aversion to medical rationing and a toleration of what elsewhere is elsewhere sometimes considered futile for economic reasons. Belgium's health-care system based on open access, free choice and fee-for-service is more likely to promote overconsumption than economy. However, like all advanced countries with an aging population Belgium faces a growing problem of funding of social security and health care. Yet, there is a dearth of studies addressing medical futility. It is as if the dominant paradigm of empowerment of individual citizens to decide for themselves discourages the performance of studies which are likely to suggest limitations on the delivery of health care. The fraction of lifelong healthcare expenditure used during the last phase of life would be expected to reduced by Belgium's high level of penetration of palliative care and to much lesser extent the availability of euthanasia. This is probably true for the former, including end-of-life decisions such as discontinuation of life-prolonging treatment and palliative sedation, but doubtful for the euthanasia. Most probably, euthanasia does not produce savings in health-care expenditure. This is because most practitioners of euthanasia agree that -statistically- cancer patients who eventually die with euthanasia tend to live longer than their counterparts dying in conventional care. The perspective of a good death at the time of choosing seems to promote serenity and a concentration on enjoyment of the last phase of life, which tends to prolong it. Also, some patients are on record to have accepted life-prolonging treatments such as brain irradiation only on the condition that they would be entitled to euthanasia if they were to develop side effects which they could not tolerate. Therefore, we see no sound foundation for the concern of opponents of euthanasia that economic motives would in the future be invoked to nudge or even coerce patients to request euthanasia.

REFERENCES

Baily MA. 2011. Futility, autonomy, and cost in end-of-life care. *Journal of Law, Medicine and Ethics* 39: 172–182.

Bassel A. 2010. Order at the end of life: Establishing a clear and fair mechanism for the resolution of futility disputes. *Vanderbilt Law Review* 63: 495–540.

Beauchamp TL and Childress JF. 1979. *Principles of Biomedical Ethics.* Oxford: Oxford University Press.

Bernheim JL. 2001. The doctor's dilemma between patient autonomy and physician beneficence at the end of life II. A-patient-physician information and communicaton covenant (ICC) as a procedural-ethical solution [in Dutch]. *Ethiek en Maatschappij* 4: 114–121.

Bernheim J. 2002. On Catholics and free-thinkers, lighthouses and navigation systems. Reflections on the euthanasia debate [in Dutch]. *Streven*, Juni: 523–537.

Bernheim JL, Deschepper R, Distelmans W, Mullie A, Bilsen J, and Deliens L. 2008. Development of palliative care and legalisation of euthanasia: Antagonism or synergy? *British Medical Journal* 336: 864–867.

Betancourt v. *Trinitas Regional Medical Hospital*, 2009, the Superior Court of New Jersey stated: "The decision to continue or terminate life support systems is not left to the courts." The appeal was dismissed by the Superior Court of New Jersey, Appellate Division 1. *Atlantic Reporter*, Third Series, No. 823, 2010.

Bilsen J, Cohen J, Chambaere K *et al.* 2009. Medical end-of-life practices under the euthanasia law in Belgium. *New England Journal of Medicine* 361: 1119–1121.

Buiting HM, Rurup ML, Wijsbek H, van Zuylen L, and den Hartogh G. 2011. Understanding provision of chemotherapy to patients with end stage cancer: qualitative interview study. *British Medical Journal* 342: d1933.

Chambaere K, Bilsen J, Cohen J, Onwuteaka-Philipsen BD, Mortier F, and Deliens L. 2010a. Physician-assisted deaths under the euthanasia law in Belgium: A population-based survey. *Canadian Medical Association Journal* 182: 895–901.

Chambaere K, Bilsen J, Cohen J, Onwuteaka-Philipsen BD, Mortier F, and Deliens L. 2010b. Trends in medical end-of-life decision making in Flanders, Belgium 1998-2001-2007. *Medical Decision Making* 31: 500–510.

Chambaere K, Centeno C, Hernández EA *et al.* 2011. *Palliative Care Development in Countries with a Euthanasia Law.* Report for the Commission on Assisted Dying Briefing Papers. Submitted October 4. Available at: http://www.commissiononassisteddying.co.uk/publications.

Court Case 1991. Court Namur 25 Octobre 1991. *Journal du Procès* No. 203, p. 26.

Delbeke E. 2012. *Juridische Aspecten van Zorgverlening aan Het Levenseinde.* Antwerp-Cambridge: Intersentia, pp. 1352–1402.

Deliens L, Mortier F, Bilsen J *et al.* 2000. End-of-life decisions in medical practice in Flanders, Belgium: A nationwide survey. *The Lancet* 356: 1806–1811.

Deschepper R, Bernheim J, Vander Stichele R *et al.* 2008. Truth-telling at the end of life: A pilot study on the perspective of patients and professional caregivers. *Patient Education and Counseling* 71: 52–56.

Downie J, Chambaere K, and Bernheim JL. 2012. Pereira's attack on legalizing euthanasia or assisted suicide: Smoke and mirrors. *Current Oncology* 13: 133–138.

Earle CC, Landrum MB, Souza JM *et al.* 2008. Aggressiveness of cancer care near the end of life: is it a quality-of-care issue?, *Journal of Clinical Oncology* 26: 3860–3866.

European Values Study. 2008. 4th wave, Integrated Dataset. GESIS Data Archive, Cologne, Germany, ZA4800 Data File Version 1.0.0 (2010-06-30) DOI:10 4232/1 10059.

Federal Advisory Committee on Bioethics. 2007. Advies nr. 41 over de geïnformeerde toestemming en DNR-codes, p. 9. Available at: www.health.belgium. be/eportal/healthcare [Accessed October 4, 2012].

FOD Volksgezondheid (Federal Government Service Public Health) Jaarstatistieken van de beoefenaars van gezondheidszorgberoepen in Belgie

2011. Available at: http://www.health.belgium.be/Healthcare/Consultative-bodies/Planningcommission/Statistiquesannuelles/12056470 [last visited Aug 5, 2012].

Genicot G. 2010. *Droit Médical et Biomédical*. Brussels: Larcier, pp. 642–654.

Gielen B, Remacle A, and Mertens R. 2010. Patterns of health care use and expenditure during the last 6 months of life in Belgium: Differences between age categories in cancer and non-cancer patients. *Health Policy* 97: 53–61.

Gomes B, Higginson IJ, Calanzani N *et al.* (on behalf of PRISMA). 2012. Preferences for place of death if faced with advanced cancer: A population survey in England, Flanders, Germany, Italy, the Netherlands, Portugal and Spain. *Annals of Oncology* 23: 2006–2015.

Gomez-Batiste X, Tuca A, Corrales E *et al.* 2006. Resource consumption and costs of palliative care services in Spain: A multicenter prospective study. *Journal of Pain and Symptom Management* 31: 522–532.

Halman LCJM. 2011. European Values Study 1999/2000, EVS '99/2000 (ZA Study 3811) (computer file). Amsterdam: Steinmetz-archief (P1460).

Ho TH, Barbera L, Saskin R, Lu H, Neville BA, and Earle CC. 2011. Trends in the aggressiveness of end-of-life cancer care in the universal health care system of Ontario, Canada. *Journal of Clinical Oncology* 29: 1587–1591.

Lantos JD, Singer PA, Walker RM *et al.* 1989. The illusion of futility in clinical practice. *The American Journal of Medicine* 87: 81–84.

Leenen H, Gevers J, and Legemaate J. 2007. *Handboek Gezondheidsrecht: Rechten van Mensen in de Gezondheidszorg*. Houten: Bohn Stafleu van Loghum, p. 321.

Lemmens C. 2012. A new style of end-of-life cases: A patient's right to demand treatment or a physician's right to refuse treatment? The futility debate revisited. Paper for the World Conference on Medical Law, Maceio (Brazil), August 2012, p. 2 (to be published in the *European Journal of Health Law*, 2012–2013).

Löfmark R and Nilstun T. 2002. Conditions and consequences of medical futility — from a literature review to a clinical model. *Journal of Medical Ethics* 28: 115–119.

Mack JW, Cronin A, Keating NL *et al.* 2012. Associations between end-of-life discussion characteristics and care received near death: A prospective cohort study. *Journal of Clinical Oncology* 30: 4387–4395.

Materstvedt LJ, Clark D, Ellershaw J *et al.* 2003. Euthanasia and physician-assisted suicide: A view from the EAPC Ethics Task Force. *Palliative Medicine* 17: 97–101.

McIntyre A. 2004. The double life of double effect. *Theoretical Medicine and Bioethics* 25: 61–74.

Medical Order. 2003. Advies van 22 maart 2003 betreffende palliatieve zorg, euthanasie en andere medische beslissingen omtrent het levenseinde. Available at: www.ordomedic.be.

Meeussen K, Van den Block L, Bossuyt N *et al.* 2009. GPs' awareness of patients' preference for place of death. *British Journal of General Practice* 59: 665–670.

Mitchell K, Kerridge I, and Lovat T. 1993. Medical futility, treatment withdrawal and the persistent vegetative state. *Journal of Medical Ethics* 19: 71–76.

Niederman MS and Berger JT. 2010. The delivery of futile care is harmful to other patients. *Critical Care Medicine* 38: S518–522.

Nys H. 2005. *Geneeskunde. Recht en Medisch Handelen.* Brussels: Story-Scientia, p. 358.

Obade C. 2011. *Patient-Care Decision-Making: A Legal Guide for Providers.* Thomson Reuters Westlaw, 10: 2.

Pardon K, Deschepper R, Vander Stichele R *et al.* 2009. Preferences of advanced lung cancer patients for patient-centred information and decision-making: A prospective multicentre study in 13 hospitals in Belgium. *Patient Education and Counseling* 77: 421–429.

Pardon K, Deschepper R, Vander Stichele R *et al.* 2010. Preferences of patients with advanced lung cancer regarding the involvement of family and others in medical decision-making. *Journal of Palliative Medicine* 13: 1199–1203.

Pardon K, Deschepper R, Vander Stichele R *et al.* 2011. Are patients' preferences for information and participation in medical decision-making being met? Interview study with lung cancer patients. *Palliative Medicine* 25: 62–70.

Pardon K, Deschepper R, Vander Stichele R *et al.* 2012a. Changing preferences for information and participation in the last phase of life: A longitudinal study among newly diagnosed advanced lung cancer patients. *Support Care Cancer* 20: 2473–2482.

Pardon K, Deschepper R, Vander Stichele R *et al.* 2012b. Preferred and actual involvement of advanced lung cancer patients and their families in end-of-life decision making: A multicenter study in 13 hospitals in Flanders, Belgium. *Journal of Pain and Symptom Management* 43: 515–526.

Paz-Ruiz S, Gómez-Batiste X *et al.* 2009. The cost and saving of a regional public palliative care program: The Catalan experience at 18 years. *Journal of Pain and Symptom Management* 38: 87–96.

Pereira J. 2011. Legalizing euthanasia or assisted suicide: The illusion of safeguards and controls. *Current Oncology* 18: e38–45.

Rietjens JA, Deschepper R, Pasman R, and Deliens L. 2012. Medical end-of-life decisions: Does its use differ in vulnerable patient groups? A systematic review and meta-analysis. *Social Science and Medicine* 74: 1282–1287.

Schneiderman LJ. 2011. Defining medical futility and improving medical care. *Journal of Bioethical Inquiry* 8: 123–131.

Smets T, Bilsen J, Cohen J, Rurup M, and Deliens L. 2010. Legal euthanasia in Belgium: Characteristics of all reported euthanasia cases. *Medical Care* 48: 187–192.

Tack S and Balthazar T. 2007. *Patiëntenrechten. Informed Consent in de Zorgsector: Recente Evoluties*. Brussels: De Boeck, p. 71.

The Law Concerning Hospitals 2008, Article 70, Law concerning hospitals 10 July 2008, BS 7 November 2008.

The Law Concerning Healthcare Professions 1967, Article 11, Law concerning healthcare professions, 10 November 1967, BS 14 November 1967.

Van den Block L, Van Casteren V, Deschepper R *et al.* 2007. Nationwide monitoring of end-of-life care via the Sentinel Network of General Practitioners in Belgium: The research protocol of the SENTI-MELC study. *BMC Palliative Care* 6: 6.

Van den Block L, Deschepper R, Bossuyt N *et al.* 2008. Care for patients in the last months of life: The Belgian Sentinel Network Monitoring End-of-Life Care study. *Archives of Internal Medicine* 168: 1747–1754.

Van den Block L, Deschepper R, Bilsen J, Bossuyt N, Van Casteren V, and Deliens L. 2009. Euthanasia and other end of life decisions and care provided in final three months of life: Nationwide retrospective study in Belgium. *BMJ* 339: b2772.

Vansweevelt T. 2003. De euthanasiewet: De ultieme bevestiging van het zelfbeschikkingsrecht of een gecontroleerde keuzevrijheid? *Tijdschrift voor Gezondheidsrecht/Revue de Droit Santé*, p. 229.

Veatch RM. 2009. The evolution of death and dying controversies. *The Hastings Center Report* 39: 16–19.

White BP, Willmott L, Ashby M. 2011. Palliative care, double effect and the law in Australia. *Internal Medical Journal* 41: 485–492.

Winkler EC, Hiddemann W, and Marckmann G. 2012. Evaluating a patient's request for life-prolonging treatment: An ethical framework. *Journal of Medical Ethics* 38: 647–651.

Youngner SJ. 1990. Futility in context. *Journal of the American Medical Association* 264: 1295–1296.

CHAPTER FOUR

THE CONCEPT OF MEDICAL FUTILITY IN VENEZUELA

Gabriel d'Empaire

SUMMARY

The development of new technologies has improved the health, life expectancy, and quality of life of many people around the world. At the same time, the diversity of new treatments has created serious doubts about the proper use of these new techniques. This is particularly true in patients at the end of life, in whom serious doubts exist about how life-sustaining interventions should either be applied or should be withheld or withdrawn. The concept of futility has been helpful in clarifying many of these situations. When a treatment is considered futile it is easier to accept the decision of withholding or withdrawing it. However, the use of the concept of futility in clinical practices has been limited because a clear definition of futility has not been possible to achieve. In this chapter, with a brief review of the healthcare system in Venezuela, I describe ethical and legal aspects of medical futility and end-of-life issues, how medical professionals deal with it, and how decisions are made in the case of futile treatment.

INTRODUCTION

The development of new diagnostic and therapeutic methods has improved the health, life expectancy, and quality of life of many people around the world. These technological advances have given us the power to help many people whose illnesses would be impossible to treat a few decades ago. At the same time, these benefits have been partially offset by many problems which have arisen as a consequence of these new technologies. One of these negative consequences is the difficulty in making the right decision about the right treatment that should be offered. The diversity of new treatments has created serious doubts about the proper use and accountability of these new techniques. This is particularly true in patients at the end of life, in whom the same treatment and technique, usually used to save lives, might just contribute to prolonging the process of dying, and increase the suffering as well as medical costs.

Therefore, serious doubts exist about how life-sustaining interventions should be applied, and when they should be withheld or withdrawn from patients with low possibility of surviving, or from patients with some chance of survival but with a limited quality of life, such as patients who suffer from advanced forms of cancer, AIDS, or are in a vegetative state.

Withholding and withdrawing medical treatments represent one of the most complex challenges we face in medical ethics. Who should be treated? Who should not be treated? How long should a patient receive treatment when he or she is not responding to the treatment properly? Which criteria must be used to make these kinds of decisions? Who is entitled to make a decision in such cases? All these questions must be answered when we deal with a patient in terminal stages. The concept of futility has been helpful in clarifying many of these situations. When a treatment is considered futile, it is more convincing to make a decision to withhold or withdraw the treatment. It should be noted that, for medical professionals in Venezuela, rationing is easier to understand when we are referring to futile treatments. However, application of the concept of futility in clinical practice has been limited, because the concept of medical futility lacks a clear definition and consensus among medical professionals. Different definitions of futility have been proposed (Schneiderman *et al.* 1990). A treatment is considered futile if it fails to achieve a specific goal. In this regard, an intervention can be simultaneously futile in achieving one goal, and quite successful in attaining another goal (Younger 1996). However, when it comes to the application of the proposed definitions, there is evidence that physicians use futility at varying degrees (Lantos *et al.* 1989; Curtis *et al.* 1995).

Reviewing the current discussion on medical futility shows that different reasons limit the use of this concept. First, in medicine, life support technology progresses faster than prognostic technology which makes it very difficult to establish the futility of some treatments. Second, in some cases it is difficult to establish the goal of the particular treatment. Third, the concept of futility is influenced by the patient's values, experience, expectations, clinical context, evidence, and medical costs. Finally, the meaning of the word "futility" is different in different languages and cultures. In this sense, in our country, Venezuela, it is more common to use the term "useless treatment" rather than "futile treatment". It is because the meaning of the word "futility" in Spanish is not the same as in English. In Spanish the word "futility" (*futilidad*) refers to something of little appreciation or little importance.

In the current situation due to the fast development of new treatments and techniques patients are more exposed to futile treatments. Any attempt to better define this concept would be helpful, and it would contribute to reduce the suffering and cost associated with the futile use of these kinds of treatments.

THE HEALTHCARE SYSTEM IN VENEZUELA

The Bolivarian Republic of Venezuela is a federal state organized into 23 federated states, a capital district, and the federal dependencies. The actual population is 28,583,000 and people under the age of 15 and above the age of 60 make up 32.1% and 7.3% of the total population, respectively. In Venezuela, life expectancy at birth is 71 years for men and 78 years for women. Gross national income per capita is 12,850 USD, total expenditure on health per capita is 275 USD, and the probability of dying under age of five (per 1,000 live births) is 18 (WHO 2011).

The healthcare system in Venezuela integrates public and private subsectors. Some healthcare facilities are also managed by the regional governments, counties, NGOs, professional and religious entities, but they cover small groups of the population. The public subsector is a free-of-charge service. According to Article 84 of the Constitution, the health system in Venezuela is "… decentralized and participatory in nature, integrated with the social security system and governed by the principles of gratuity, universality, completeness, fairness, social integration …" (Bolivarian Republic of Venezuela Constitution 1999). The same Article of the Constitution establishes the creation of a National Public Health System. The National Law of Health to regulate this National Public Health System is being discussed at the National Assembly, and it will substitute the actual National Law of Health of 1998 (National Law of Health 1998).

The Health Ministry of Popular Power created the National Plan of Health (NPH) 2009–2013/2018 (Ministry of Popular Power for Health 2010). The main goal of the NPH is to warrant the quality of life and health of the individual citizens, consolidating the National Public Health System, by following the constitutional mandate, and having the Misión Barrio Adentro (Inside the Neighborhood Mission) as the main axis of medical care.

The Misión Barrio Adentro began in 2001 as an ambulatory level of an integral healthcare strategy, to improve the efficacy of the first level of healthcare. However, structural changes were made to the healthcare system, and the Misión Barrio Adentro was formally created on May 22, 2003. The main objective was to increase the coverage of basic health services with quality and equity.

The Misión Barrio Adentro has different levels: Barrio Adentro I was created as the primary level of healthcare. The main aspect of these centers is that they are located in the neighborhoods and in the marginalized areas of the large cities, although some facilities were located in higher-income areas. The second level of healthcare, Barrio Adentro II, focuses on secondary care in three main areas: Integral Diagnostic Areas, Rehabilitation Integral Areas, and High Technology Centers.

The third level of healthcare, Barrio Adentro III, provides care for those cases which cannot be resolved at the two lower levels. This level is made up of 220 hospitals with complex healthcare facilities which provide care to referral patients from the first and second levels.

Barrio Adentro IV is in charge of the most complicated and specialized medical and surgical needs.

The private sector charges a fee for service, some institutions are for profit, and others are non-profit health organizations. The cost of medical care is usually covered by private insurance, and only in a few cases, the payment is covered by the patient. Each person is free to decide if they want to obtain personal insurance. Part of the medical costs of an insured patient is paid by the employers. However, a significant part of the population has no economic capacity to pay for insurance policies. In the past few years, the number of people insured by the government has increased (PROVEA 2010), and as a consequence the number of patients consulting private hospitals has increased.

Currently, there is no data available to evaluate how the payment system affects decision making about medical futility. The use of futile treatments usually does not depend on the payment system. Obviously, in a free-of-charge public healthcare system there is less pressure to use futile treatments than in a private system. However, the medical indications are made by medical doctors, and there is no strict control by the hospital's administration, either in the public or the private hospitals, regarding the type of medical treatment.

MEDICAL FUTILITY AND END-OF-LIFE: WHO DECIDES AND HOW?

The first relevant aspect that we have in Venezuela regarding ethics at the end of life comes from Dr. Luis Razetti, a Venezuelan medical doctor born in 1862. He was a pioneer in medical ethics in our country and in South America. He wrote the first ethical code in medicine in Venezuela, and also was the author of Razetti's Oath which is still used at the Universidad Central de Venezuela to confirm the commitment required for all medical doctors who receive a medical degree from this University (Razetti 1928). In this oath Dr. Razetti said: "My reverence for the life when I treat terminal patients will not compete with my fundamental obligation to relieve human suffering." So, according to Dr. Razetti we can understand that to treat human suffering is more important than the life itself (Aguiar-Guevara 2001). Furthermore, it is important to highlight that our Medical Code of Ethics (Medical Deontology Code 2004) establishes in Article 84 that "… to relieve suffering is a fundamental medical obligation and under no circumstances the doctor may deliberately provoke the patient's death even if their families request it". In other words active euthanasia is expressly prohibited.

In our country, with the exception of active euthanasia, the management of patients at the end of life has different approaches. In this regard, there is not, as perhaps in many other countries, a clear ethical framework in relation to the protocol to be followed in such cases. Physicians, the health staff, patients, their families, and society in general face the issue of the end of life with different criteria, depending on their values, religion, information, and expectations. In this sense, we can find extremes, from those who advocate active euthanasia to those who, even in terminal situations, do not accept any means to shorten the life, or any form of limitation of treatments even when they might be futile. However, the majority accept the limits of medical care, and when the patient is considered irrecoverable, measures are taken to respect the patient's rights and dignity, and to reduce the risk of using futile treatments.

A study conducted to evaluate physicians' opinions about decisions at the end of life revealed that 85% of the physicians agreed to withhold or withdraw medical treatments in a terminal patient and just 3% of them disagreed. The majority (85%) were opposed to the admission of these terminal patients to intensive care units and 5% approved of the admission of those patients. Ten percent of the respondents did not answer this question. Sixty-four percent of the physicians refused to use medical treatments which could prolong the life of a terminal patient. The majority (82%) considered that, if the patients didn't have the capacity, the decision had to be made by the family members along with the physician and the critical care unit staff. However, there still remained 14% of physicians who thought that this kind of decision should exclude the family members.

Fifty percent of the physicians consulted would continue with all treatments, even when they could be considered futile, if the patient or the family members insisted on continuing the life-sustaining treatment. Of them, 39% refused to continue futile treatments and preferred to refer the patient to another doctor; 11% did not answer.

The study showed that the majority of respondents (57%) believed that cost was an element to take into account when deciding about the limitation of therapeutic measures and 36% did not consider it an important factor in decision making.

In that study, 94% of the physicians considered that all competent patients had the right to know their medical situation and should participate in any decisions about their treatments. Most doctors (97%) agreed that the patients had the right to refuse receiving certain treatments. Of them, 77% believed that physicians should not give treatments against the patient's will. Of the respondents, 83% believed that it was important to take into account the opinion of other health team members when a decision to withhold or withdraw treatment had to be made. They also considered unanimity important in this kind of decision (d'Empaire *et al.* 2002).

In another study to evaluate different aspects of withholding and withdrawing medical treatment, we found that in 85.7% of the cases, the decision was discussed with the patient's family members. In 77.7% of these patients the family actively participated. However, 7.49% of the family members, after receiving the information, preferred not to participate in the decision and accepted the physician's proposal. In 14.29% of cases the family members did not participate, and the decision was taken by the medical doctors. In this study, 100% of the patients had no capacity to make their own decision and none of them had a living will. In 34.92% of the patients, treatments were withheld, and in 65.98% treatments were withdrawn. Treatment futility was the reason for withholding or withdrawing treatments in 100% of the cases. In this study, the cost of medical care was not considered a reason for the decision making (d'Empaire *et al.* 2001).

These two studies reflect the ethical trend in end-of-life decision making in our country. Although differences still exist, in most cases the decisions are taken after long deliberation, in which healthcare providers consider the patient's diagnosis and prognosis, to ensure that the patient is in the terminal stage. However, to reduce harm, the effectiveness of possible medical indications is discussed in order to avoid the use of futile treatments, which could needlessly prolong the dying process, increasing the patient's suffering and medical costs. Finally, in order to respect the principle of autonomy, as well as the patient's dignity and rights, in most cases the patient's wishes (or the surrogate's opinion when the patient has no capacity) are taken into account in decision making.

MEDICAL FUTILITY: RELATED LEGISLATION AND GUIDELINES

There are no specific laws, guidelines, professional codes, or protocols to regulate medical futility in Venezuela. However, the Constitution and other laws regulate different aspects regarding healthcare at the end of life which can be applicable in the case of medical futility. The Constitution of the Bolivarian Republic of Venezuela (Bolivarian Republic of Venezuela Constitution 1999) was approved in 1999 by a popular referendum. It was adopted in December 1999, and it replaced the previous Constitution of 1961. Different articles refer to the protection of human rights, the right to life, the right to health, and the right to be informed. For example, Article 19 reads:

"The State shall guarantee to every individual, in accordance with the progressive principle and without discrimination of any kind, not renounceable, indivisible and interdependent enjoyment and exercise of human rights. Respect for and the guaranteeing of these rights is obligatory for the organs of Public Power, in accordance with the Constitution, the human rights treaties signed and ratified by the Republic and any laws developing the same."

Article 43 protects the right to life. It reads: "The right to life is inviolable. No law shall provide for the death penalty and no authority shall apply the same. The State shall protect the life of persons who are deprived of liberty, serving in the armed forces or civilian services, or otherwise subject to its authority."

Articles 83, 84, and 85 recognize and guarantee the right to health as a fundamental social right as part of the right to life. Article 83 says:

"Health is a fundamental social right and the responsibility of the State, which shall guarantee it as part of the right to life. The State shall promote and develop policies oriented toward improving the quality of life, common welfare and access to services. All persons have the right to protection of health, as well as the duty to participate actively in the furtherance and protection of the same..."

According to Article 84, "In order to guarantee the right to health, the State creates, exercises guidance over and administers a national public health system that crosses sector boundaries, and is decentralized and participatory in nature, integrated with the social security system and governed by the principles of gratuity, universality, completeness, fairness, social integration and solidarity."

The Constitution also establishes informed consent. As Article 46 reads: "Everyone is entitled to respect for his or her physical, mental and moral integrity, therefore: (3) No person shall be subjected without his or her freely given consent to scientific experiments or medical or laboratory examinations, except when such person's life is in danger, or in any other circumstances as may be detained by law."

The National Law of Health of 1998 establishes the right of terminal patients to refuse extraordinary treatments. According to Article 69 patients have the following rights:

- Respect for their dignity and privacy, and cannot be discriminated against because of geographical, racial, social, sexual, economical, ideological, political or religious reasons.
- To accept or refuse to participate, after receiving information, in research projects.
- To receive information, in understandable terms, with regard to health and treatment of their disease, in order to give informed consent to the diagnostic and therapeutic options, unless epidemic risks of severe or extreme urgency exist.
- To refuse extraordinary treatments addressed to prolong their life when, according to the state of the art in medicine, they are in the terminal stage.

It should be noted that the Law of Medicine (1982) considers no obligation for using measures to artificially sustain life in terminal patients and also regulates the admission or stay of terminal patients in intensive care units. Article 28 reads: "The doctor treating not recoverable patients has no obligation to use extraordinary measures to maintain artificial life. In these cases, if possible, hear the opinion of another or other medical professionals. Regulations will develop the content of this provision."

According to Article 29, "The admission and stay of patients in intensive care units should be subject to strict evaluation, designed to prevent the unjustified, useless and expensive use of these services in conditions in which they are not needed or in case of care of patients irrecoverable at the final stage of their illness."

The Medical Deontology Code

The Medical Deontology Code, approved in October 2004 by the CXL Venezuelan Medical Federation Assembly, has a level of law. Regarding end-of-life decision making, this Code states in Article 77 that "The patients with a terminal illness have the right to be informed of the truth of their condition, if they want to know it. The physician must make the preliminary assessment of these patients to determine the appropriate time to provide the required information and has to be prepared to assist the patient in case of unpredictable reactions." Article 78 of this Code says: "Patients in a terminal condition and who are mentally competent have the right to participate in decisions about their illness, for which they should be properly informed about the available options, possible benefits or adverse effects which could be related to them. The patient may refuse any diagnostic or therapeutic procedure and his or her decision must be respected."

If the treatment is believed to be futile, according to this Code (Article 82), terminally ill patients should not be subjected to measures derived from life support technology, which only serve to prolong the agony but do not preserve life.

Article 83 says:

"When a terminally ill patient is suffering from pain, the physician should use analgesics in sufficient doses to relieve suffering if it is necessary for the physician to carry out therapeutic measures to relieve pain. In those cases where a gradual increase in the dose of strong painkillers can shorten the life by depression of the center that regulates breathing, the physician should give priority to the analgesic treatment as a primary effect wanted."

Article 84 of this Code sets the primary obligation for physicians to relieve human suffering. They cannot deliberately provoke the patient's death, under any circumstances, even if he or his family requests it, nor shall either cooperate or assist in the suicide of the patient by procuring a drug in a lethal dose.

THE LINK BETWEEN MEDICAL FUTILITY AND EUTHANASIA

Although in Venezuela medical futility is applicable in medical practice, active euthanasia is expressly prohibited. Therefore, it is not possible to relate the concept of medical futility to active euthanasia.

For a patient in the terminal stage of illness, attempts to define the effectiveness or futility of treatments are usually made. In this sense, our laws clearly establish the terminal patient's right to be informed of the truth of their condition; the right to participate in decisions about their illness; the right to be properly informed about the available options, possible benefits, or adverse effects which could be related to them; and the right to refuse any diagnostic or therapeutic procedure which prolong their life if according to the state of the art in medicine, the patient is in the terminal stage. It should be noted that the Penal Code of Venezuela prohibits the assistance of suicide. Some proposals have been made to include articles to permit euthanasia, but those articles have not been approved.

The law of medicine also establishes no obligation for using measures to artificially sustain life if there is no possibility of recovery. In Venezuela, in order to prevent the use of scarce resources and health services, in case of futile treatment and irrecoverable patients, there is a strict evaluation of admissions or stays in intensive care units to see if they are unjustified, useless, and expensive. In other words, this law prohibits the use of futile treatments.

CONCLUSION

Despite the advances in medical sciences, our capacity to sustain life with a reasonable quality of life in patients who suffer from irrecoverable illnesses is limited. In this regard, any attempt to better define the concept of medical futility in clinical practice, as well as advances in improving our capacity to establish the patient's prognosis and the guarantee to respect the patient's right to be informed and their right to make their own decision based on their values, will improve our quality of healthcare, reduce the patients' suffering, and reduce medical costs. In clinical practice in Venezuela, the tendency is to prevent the use of futile treatments at the end of life. This tendency is clearly expressed in the studies mentioned earlier in this article (d'Empaire *et al.* 2002), where 85% of the physicians agreed with withholding or withdrawing medical treatment if it is futile in terminal patients, and only 3% of them disagreed with this procedure. The majority (85%) were opposed to the admission of these terminal patients to intensive care units; 64% of the physicians refused to use medical treatments which could prolong the life of terminal patients. However, 50% of the physicians consulted would continue with all treatments, even when they could be considered futile, if the patient or the family members insisted on continuing the treatment.

REFERENCES

Aguiar-Guevara R. 2001. *Tratado de Derecho Médico*. Caracas: Legis Editores, p. 625.

Bolivarian Republic of Venezuela Constitution 1999. Available at: http://axiso-flogic.com/artman/publish/Article_29889.shtml [Accessed May 15, 2012].

Curtis JR, Park DR, Krone MR *et al.* 1995. Use of the medical futility rationale in do not attempt resuscitation orders. *JAMA* 273: 124–128.

d'Empaire G, Parada MI, d'Empaire MA, and Encinoso J. 2001. Limitación de medidas terapéuticas en pacientes hospitalizados en una unidad de cuidados intensivos. *Clínica Médica HCC* 6: 143–146.

d'Empaire G, Parada MI, d'Empaire MA, and Encinoso J. 2002. Limitación de medidas terapéuticas: Opinión de médicos de diversas especialidades. *Clínica Médica HCC* 7: 29–36.

Lantos JD, Singer PA, Walker PM *et al.* 1989. The illusion of futility in clinical practice. *American Journal of Medicine* 87: 81–84.

Law of Medicine. Available at: http://legal.com.ve/leyes/C106.pdf [Accessed May 15, 2012].

Medical Deontology Code of 2004. Available at: http://www.saber.ula.ve/bitstream/123456789/32938/8/5ta_sesion_codigoetica.pdf.

Ministry of Popular Power for Health. 2010. *Memoria 2010*. Available at: http://www.ovsalud.org/doc/Memoria_2010.pdf [Accessed June 20, 2011].

National Law of Health 1998. Available at: http://www.derechos.org.ve/pw/ wpcontent/uploads/ley_organica_salud.pdf [Accessed May 15, 2012].

PROVEA. 2010. *Informe Anual.* Available at: http://www.derechos.org.ve/ informes-anuales/informe-anual-2010/.

Razetti L. 1928. Razetti's Oath. Available at: http://antonio7635.wordpress. com/2008/06/09/juramento-de-razetti/ [Accessed May 15, 2012].

Schneiderman L, Jecker NS, and Jonsen AR. 1990. Medical futility: Its meaning and ethical implications. *Annals of Internal Medicine* 112: 949–954.

World Health Organization. 2011. Venezuela: Health profile. Available at: http:// www.who.int/gho/countries/ven.pdf [Accessed June 20, 2011].

Younger S. 1996. Medical futility. In: KA Koch, ed. *Medical Ethics. Critical Care Clinics.* Philadelphia: WB Saunders Company, Vol. 12, pp. 165–178.

CHAPTER FIVE

MEDICAL FUTILITY IN THE RUSSIAN FEDERATION

Olga I Kubar, Galina L Mikirtichian
and Marina I Petrova

SUMMARY

In the Russian Federation the term "futile medicine" is absent from the vocabulary of medical professionals, and therefore medical futility is considered in the context of palliative medicine. The entire history of medicine in Russia, starting from the nineteenth century, shows that the work of Russian physicians and their practice has been focused on relieving terminal illness, providing merciful care and maintaining, to the maximum extent possible, the quality of the patient's life with regard to any stage of a terminal illness. Since the end of the twentieth century, there have been positive results in the development of a regulatory and administrative framework for palliative care in Russia. One of the positive results is the recognition of the importance of ethical and legal regulation in palliative medicine with regard to human rights, the value of human life, the protection of human rights and freedoms. Further development of ethics and law in the field of palliative medicine in Russia can be facilitated by legislative initiatives in the sphere of human rights, continuous work on adaptation and implementation of international rules, regulations and administrative procedures for providing medical care in the case of medical futility.

THE HEALTHCARE SYSTEM IN THE RUSSIAN FEDERATION

The healthcare system of the Russian Federation is a complex of federal health agencies, the executive board, executive agencies, local authorities and their subordinate organizations, as well as institutions of private medical practice and private pharmaceutical activity. Their responsibility is to protect and strengthen the health of citizens. All structural elements of the system are enshrined in the relevant legislation. In accordance with the Fundamentals of the Russian Federation Legislation on Citizens' Health Protection (Fundamentals 2011), and depending on the form of property and funding sources, there are three healthcare systems in the Russian Federation: state, municipal and private medical system.

The state healthcare system includes federal agencies of executive power, the executive authorities of the Russian Federation, institutions of the Russian Academy of Medical Sciences, as well as state-owned institutions for preventive medicine, research, education, pharmacy and public health.

The municipal healthcare system comprises local government bodies authorized to exercise control in medical and pharmaceutical organizations owned by municipalities.

The private healthcare system includes medical and pharmaceutical institutions whose property is owned by the private sector, as well as professionals engaged in private medical practice and private pharmaceutical activities.

Institutions in the healthcare system in Russia provide various kinds of medical care. There are several classifications of medical care: primary healthcare, emergency and specialized medical care, and medical and social assistance to citizens suffering from social diseases and individuals suffering from diseases that present a danger to others. The most high-volume type of care is primary healthcare (PHC), which is available free of charge for every citizen.

Depending on the stage of rendering medical care there are different levels of healthcare delivery: first, secondary and tertiary healthcare.

According to the Russian Federation Healthcare Ministry Order in 2005, there are different district, city, regional and republican hospitals as well as specialized hospitals for certain diseases such as cancer, geriatric, psycho-neurological and psychiatric hospitals for both children and adult patients.

The nomenclature includes also nursing homes, hospices, as well as dispensaries of different profiles. District and city outpatient clinics provide medical services to children and adults. There are also some special healthcare institutions dealing with specific issues such as natural disaster medicine, licensing medical and pharmacy practice, quality control and certification of medicinal products, as well as the bureau of medical statistics and forensic examination, control and analytical laboratories, military medical commissions and an agency for the supervision of consumer rights protection and human welfare.

In Russia, the health insurance system has two basic services: compulsory health insurance and voluntary health insurance. Compulsory health insurance is provided by the state for social protection of citizens' interests in healthcare and covers healthcare costs. Compensation comes from resources accumulated in the compulsory health insurance funds (at the territorial and federal level). Voluntary health insurance provides insurance in case of sickness and offers an opportunity for full or partial reimbursement of medical expenses and loss of income during the illness in addition to the healthcare system or compulsory health insurance. The compulsory health insurance fund is formed from employers' insurance premiums, as well as payments from the budget for the non-working population. This insurance guarantees medical care, in the extent and on the conditions stated in the compulsory health insurance programs. This service is provided to all citizens of the Russian Federation, irrespective of sex, age, place of residence and social status. Among compulsory health insurance programs is the territorial program defining the guaranteed scope of free medical care funded by compulsory health insurance.

PALLIATIVE CARE MEDICINE IN RUSSIA

In Russia, all ethical, social, legal and medical aspects associated with end-of-life treatment are expressed through the concept of palliative medicine. These are the main characteristics of the Russian healthcare system that form the background for the development, structure and practice of palliative medicine in the country. Palliative medicine is presented in this review because the term "futile medicine" is absent from the vocabulary of the professional medical community, clinical as well as scientific, and therefore medical futility is considered in terms of palliative medicine. Further development of palliative medicine in Russia may help to introduce more precise wording for terms and concepts used by the international medical community so that we can speak the same language and discuss patient care.

Palliative medicine in Russia originated in the system of cancer care, and its concepts go back to the beginning of the twentieth century. In 1903, at the initiative of Prof. A.L. Levshina, the Morozov Institute for Tumor Treatment opened at the Medical Faculty of Moscow State University (now I.M. Sechenov First Moscow State Medical University). The Morozov Institute had a hospital for 130 inpatients, experimental and chemical laboratories, a radiology department and a laboratory for studying the effect of radioactive substances on body tissues.

In 1911, in St. Petersburg, a famous merchant Yeliseev initiated the foundation of the Yeleninskaya Hospital for 90 patients, for "poor women of Christian faiths suffering from malignant tumors". In 1908, the All-Russia Society for Cancer Control was formed in St. Petersburg. The Society opened a hospital for free treatment of cancer patients with X-rays and radium, and in 1914 convened the First All-Russia Congress on Cancer in St. Petersburg.

Later in the twentieth century, in Russia, like in other countries, the problems of cancer treatment and prevention became an issue of state concern, as proclaimed at a special meeting of the People's Commissariat for Healthcare of the Russian Soviet Federative Socialist Republic in 1925. From 1989 to 1991 the development of palliative care for cancer patients suffering from chronic pain was started. The infrastructure began to form, including pain-relief units within cancer research institutes and cancer clinics. In several cities, hospices were set up in analogy with those in Great Britain. The first Russian hospice opened in St. Petersburg in the autumn of 1990 due to the efforts of St. Petersburg psychiatrist Andrey Gnezdilov and British journalist Victor Zorza. Great support was rendered by British physicians and nurses who held a number of courses on palliative care which were extremely helpful. Currently, this hospice is a state charitable institution providing medical, psychosocial and spiritual care for terminal cancer patients, as well as family support. In 1994, the first

Moscow hospice began work. It is worth mentioning that all hospices in Russia get financial and administrative support from the government (Gnezdilov *et al.* 1994).

A hospice is defined as a medical institution providing palliative care to patients with advanced terminal cancer at the inpatient unit or at home, as well as offering psychological support to the patient's family during the illness and after the patient's death.

Currently, Russia has a network of inpatient and outpatient clinics for palliative care. Hospices and palliative medicine departments within multi-profile hospitals are mostly state owned and the services are free of charge. Besides, there are also private nursing homes, some of which provide care for elderly cancer patients. Cancer patients may receive ambulatory treatment at pain relief wards. There are also home care teams visiting cancer patients at their homes. Palliative care is rendered not only to cancer patients, but also to patients suffering from other terminal diseases such as AIDS. Alongside hospice care for adults, there is also pediatric hospice care. Hospices as well as the palliative care departments within multi-profile hospitals are financed by the state.

The practice of palliative medicine in the Russian Federation is regulated by a number of administrative documents, particularly the Recommendations for the Organization of Palliative Care developed and approved at the national level, and the Hospice Statute. The first legal document regulating palliative medicine was approved in 1992, which has stimulated the setting up of hospices, nursing homes and wards. Besides, in 1995, the status of the geriatric medical specialty was introduced. In 1996, palliative care in Russia was included in *Index Medicus*, termed "palliative care" in addition to the existing definitions of "terminal care" (1968) and "hospice" (1980). However, meanwhile, palliative medicine as a specialty is not included in the Nomenclature of Medical Specialties. All these initiatives were carried out under the auspices of the Ministry of Health of the Russian Federation.

Departments of palliative medicine are set up within cancer clinics to provide palliative care and to create conditions that ensure an optimal quality of life for cancer patients. The Program for Strategic Development of Hospice and Palliative Medicine in the Russian Federation is setting clear objectives, tasks and time frames.

The problem of opioid analgesic availability for pain relief in cancer patients should also be a subject of legislative regulation. Incurable cancer patients fall into the category of citizens who are entitled to receive a set of social services.

Another important development is the public movement supporting palliative medicine. In 1993, the Expert Council for the Organization of Palliative Care for Cancer Patients was established, followed by the creation of the Palliative Medicine and Rehabilitation of Patients Fund in 1995, which stimulated the All-Russia public movement "Medicine for Quality of Life" in 2002. The Fund's resources were used to organize conferences and provide education in dealing with patients for whom medical treatment is futile. In 1996, the *Journal of Palliative Care and Rehabilitation* was published. In 2007, an inter-regional public organization called the Association for Palliative Medicine was established in St. Petersburg.

International cooperation plays a significant role in the development of palliative care in the Russian Federation. At present, we have continuous cooperation and interaction with a number of international organizations (the European Association for Palliative Care (EAPC) and the International Association for Hospice and Palliative Care (IAHPC)). Within the framework of international cooperation, annual events, such as the celebration World Hospice and Palliative Care Day, are held.

Education in the field of palliative medicine is following. Although the specialty palliative medicine is not included in the Nomenclature of Medical Specialties of the Russian Federation Ministry of Health and Social Development, courses on palliative medicine and palliative oncology have been developed and held within the framework of postgraduate medical education. An essential contribution to postgraduate training in this field was scientific monographs and guidelines by Russian authors (Modnikov *et al.* 2004; Novikov *et al.* 2002–2003, 2004; Novikov 2000–2006).

The courses are based on the Program of Postgraduate Professional Education on Palliative Care in Oncology approved by the Russian Federation Health Ministry in 2000. The priorities of the courses are teaching, methodical and research work.

ETHICS OF END-OF-LIFE CARE IN RUSSIA

Palliative care for dying patients rests on the traditions of Russian philosophical and religious thought, on classical medical ethics, on principles and rules of bioethics and on extensive practical experience in medicine. Based on this approach, physicians should respect the patient's integrity, act in the patient's best interests and approach each patient individually considering the patient's condition, the patient's preferences, as well as therapeutic goals and benefit from each particular treatment and the side effects. This means that the physician treats the patient within reasonable limits and is aware of the natural processes of life and death. There are no objective criteria to stop the special treatment and each patient is unique. However, when treating a patient with terminal cancer it is important to see when would be proper to change to comprehensive palliative treatment, which means medical, psychosocial and spiritual care (Ekkert 2006).

Ethical principles form an essential element of the physician's practice. Symptom control does not aim at curing the terminal cancer patient; it aims at relieving or eliminating symptoms, minimizing the patient's suffering and maximizing the quality of life. A caring attitude helps the patient to go through the psychological experience and stages of coping with terminal illness to the last stage when the individual begins to come to terms with her/his mortality. This may be achieved in the atmosphere of a trustful and honest relationship between the patient and the medical professionals.

Bad news about the terminal illness and prognosis can result in depression in the patient. Therefore, for a long time the dominant deontological position was to conceal the truth from the patient and not to tell him/her about the possible fatal outcome. However, many patients with terminal cancer are aware of their illness or receive traumatic information from somewhere else. Deficient verbal information in combination with the unspoken oppressive sorrows of relatives and avoidant behavior of the medical staff negatively affected the patient's condition, and undermined the trust in medical professionals and medicine in general, which hindered effective treatment. Therefore, now the attitude is different. The patients receive truthful information, and the problem is not "to tell or not to tell", but how to tell and how to choose appropriate psychological approaches to breaking bad news in each particular case. The patient has the right to get adequate and reliable information about the illness, suggested treatment and the likely prognosis, as well as emotional support on the way towards accepting the approaching death. The patient has the right to choose how to use the remaining time of his/her life (to arrange his/her personal and family affairs, to change his/her way of life or to refuse both the information about his/her conditions and the proposed treatment, etc.).

Informed voluntary consent is a rule in the relationship with the patient and/or his legal representatives, as stipulated by the Russian legislation on healthcare. Medical professionals should not stop therapy at the bedside of the dying patient until the patient voluntarily expresses his/her competent informed decision about the termination of active medical treatment and transition to palliative care or refuse the therapy altogether. The change in treatment procedure without the patient's consent may happen only if the patient is in a coma, in a persistent vegetative state or has mental deterioration that does not allow him/her to make an informed decision.

In Russian society, the family plays an important role in providing care for the chronically ill, which reduces the load on the organization of medical and social assistance. In the context of palliative care, family support is an integral part of caring for the dying patient. However, the family should get adequate psychological and social support, so that the patient and his/her relatives can live as fully as possible. Communication with family members aims at helping the family to cope with the impending death and bereavement.

In palliative medicine, physicians play an important role in the patient-centered team. The patient's quality of life in many respects depends on their professional qualities, communication skills and empathy. The physician's work in palliative medicine is a special type of medical activity. Physicians are facing the pain, suffering and death of their patients, and often are in situations where they have to make adequate decisions within a limited time. No wonder that burnout syndrome is a serious problem for the physicians and nurses working in this field.

The importance of nursing care cannot be overstressed. The concept of a nurse as a "sister of mercy" has been accepted as a professional standard of behavior in Russia since the days of famous Russian physician Nikolai Pirogov (19th c.) (Ivanjushkin and Hetagurova 2003).

In our days the Russian Federation Code of Ethics for Nurses states ethical rules guiding behavior towards a dying patient. This Code states, in particular: "The nurse must respect the right of the dying patient to a kind, empathic attitude and a dignified death." It also says:

"The nurse should possess the necessary knowledge and skills in palliative care, which would allow them to provide comfort and relief for the dying patient. The essential tasks of a medical nurse is to prevent or relieve sufferings associated with the process of dying and to give the dying patient and his/her family psychological support. ... Euthanasia, i.e. intentional action for terminating the patient's life, even at the patient's request, is immoral and unacceptable."

MEDICAL FUTILITY AND EUTHANASIA

Palliative care advocates the patient's right to a "good death", and the distinction between passive and active euthanasia and natural death can be very vague in the context of palliative care (Zil'ber 1998, 2002). Nevertheless, the philosophy of palliative medicine states that the deliberate termination of a patient's life is never necessary. In the case of futile treatment, palliative care is recognized as an alternative to euthanasia for terminally ill patients experiencing suffering. Doctors and nurses should understand that their duty is to sustain life, and not to promote the idea to patients of killing themselves or hastening the onset of death.

It should be especially mentioned that in matters of life and death, ethics, law and religion are closely intertwined and interrelated in Russian society. Today there is every possibility for the church institutions to promote their viewpoints on a wide range of purely secular issues — from politics, culture, science and education to ethnic and international relations (Jubilee Bishops' Council of the Russian Orthodox Church 2002).

It is well known that euthanasia is condemned by traditional religion and morality. The Ecclesiastical and Public Council for Biomedical Ethics (1999) states that "the Orthodox clergy, scientists and physicians consider euthanasia as an action of killing a terminally ill patient and also consider euthanasia as a special form of homicide (by doctors), or as a suicide (at the request of the patient), or as a combination of both" (Silujanova 2001).

The Bases of the Social Concept of the Russian Orthodox Church — the document adopted at the Jubilee Bishops' Council (2000) in the chapter "Challenges of Bioethics" — considers the problem of euthanasia, the "right to die", in terms of Christian doctrine:

> "... the Church, while remaining faithful to God's commandment 'thou shalt not kill' (Ex. 20:13), cannot recognize as morally acceptable the widely-spread attempt to legalise the so-called euthanasia, that is, the purposeful destruction of hopelessly ill patients (also by their own will). The request of a patient to speed up his death is sometimes associated with depression preventing him from assessing his condition correctly. Legalised euthanasia would lead to the devaluation of the dignity and the corruption of the professional duty of the doctor called to preserve rather than end life. 'The right to death' can easily become a threat to the life of a patient whose treatment is hampered by lack of funds. Therefore, euthanasia is considered a form of homicide or suicide, depending on whether a patient participates in it or not. Both a purposeful suicide and assistance in it are viewed as grave sins."

In general, these principles of moral behavior by medical professionals are not new; they have been followed as generally accepted standards of medical practice, which are reflected in many literary and art works by Russian authors.

END-OF-LIFE: RELATED LEGISLATION AND REGULATIONS

As mentioned earlier, in Russia the issue of medical futility has been dealt in the context of end-of-life palliative medicine. Legislative regulation of issues related to end-of-life issues are an essential component in terms of respect for human rights and interests and human dignity at all stages of life.

According to the Constitution of the Russian Federation, "Man, his rights and freedoms shall be the supreme value." The Constitution determines the full range of civil rights and freedoms. "The Russian Federation recognizes and guarantees the rights and freedoms of citizens according to the universally recognized principles and norms of international law and according to the present Constitution" (Article 17, Clause 1); "Fundamental human rights and freedoms are inalienable and shall be enjoyed by everyone from the day of birth" (Chapter 2, Article 17, Clause 2). According to Article 20, "Everyone shall have the right to life." Article 21, Clause 1 states: "Human dignity shall be protected by the State. Nothing may serve as a basis for its derogation." Article 21, Clause 2 reads: "No one shall be subject to torture, violence or other cruel or humiliating treatment or punishment. No one may be subject to medical, scientific and other experiments without voluntary consent." According to Article 22, "Everyone shall have the right to freedom and personal immunity." Article 23, Clause 1 states: "Everyone shall have the right to the inviolability of private life, personal and family secrets, the protection of one's honour and good name." Article 24 guarantees confidentiality: "The collection, keeping, use and dissemination of information about the private life of a person shall not be allowed without his or her consent" (Clause 1). "The bodies of state authority and local self-government, their officials shall ensure for everyone the possibility of acquainting themselves with the documents and materials directly affecting his or her rights and freedoms, unless otherwise provided for by law" (Clause 2).

In terms of decision making, Articles 5, 6, 13, 20 and 22 of the Fundamentals of the Russian Federation Legislation on Citizens' Health Protection (2011) describe regulations of the general character and establish the key requirements for the procedure of decision making on the nature and extent of treatment of the patient (including the dying patient).

To maintain the priority of the patient's best interests by observing ethical and moral principles, Article 6 of the Fundamentals states that in seeking and receiving medical treatment the patient has the right to respectful and considerate care by medical staff, and for his/her condition and also his/her cultural and religious traditions to be considered whenever possible. Accordingly, patients have the right to choose their physician, including the family and attending physician and healthcare facility, in compliance with the compulsory or voluntary health insurance contract. They also have the right to access to consultation with other medical specialists, access to pain relief associated with the disease and/or medical intervention by available means (the latter is of extreme importance in the case of medical futility), and the right to see a lawyer or other legal representatives to defend his/her rights, as well as a priest. It says that the hospital is responsible for providing the conditions for religious practices, including the provision of a separate room if it does not violate the internal rules of the hospital.

Article 6 also stipulates that medical institutions should create conditions for the patient's relatives to visit him/her and stay with the patient considering his/her condition. Article 22 of the Fundamentals enshrines the right of citizens to obtain information about their health. Every citizen has the right to receive information about his/her health explained in an accessible form, including information about examination results, the presence of the disease, diagnosis and prognosis, treatment options, associated risks, possible options of medical interventions and their impact on the outcome of therapy. Considering cases of patients who are legally acknowledged incapable, the Article stipulates that their legal representatives (appointed legal representatives, attending physician, the head of the department of medical and preventive treatment or other professionals directly involved in the examination and treatment) can make the decision. Since the information about diagnosis, prognosis and treatment prospects may have serious psychological and moral effects, Article 22 states also that health information cannot be enforced upon the patient against his/her will. In cases of poor prognosis of the disease, information should be delivered in a delicate way to the patient and his/her family (spouse, children, adoptees, adoptive parents, siblings, grandchildren, grandparents), if the patient has no objection to telling them about it, and/ or if he/she has not appointed a person to whom this information should be delivered.

In compliance with Article 20, the necessary precondition for a medical intervention is the citizen's (or his/her legal representative's) voluntary informed consent based on information given by the medical professional in a clear and accessible form about treatment options, associated risks, possible options of medical interventions and their impact on the outcome of therapy. If patients are recognized to be incapable, according to the legal procedure, to give their free and voluntary consent to medical intervention, it should be obtained from their legal representatives informed as stated in Article 20. In the absence of legal representatives, the medical council can make the decision about a medical intervention; if it is impossible to call the council, then the attending physician (physician on call) makes the decision with subsequent notification to the officials of the medical institution and legal representatives. The same article (Article 20) of the Fundamentals describes also essential legal situations defining the possibility and conditions to refuse a medical intervention. Accordingly, the patient or his/her legal representative has the right to refuse a medical intervention or require it to stop. In the case of refusal, the physician is obliged to explain in an accessible form all the possible consequences of renouncing medical intervention to the patient. If the patient still wants to refuse the treatment, his renunciation should be documented in writing and signed by the patient (or his/her legal representative) and the physician. However, if one of the parents or other legal representative of a patient specified in Part 2 of this Article, or a legal representative of a patient recognized as incapable according to the legal procedure, refuses life-saving medical intervention, the medical organization has the right to go to court to protect the patient's interests.

The Law on the Fundamentals of the Citizens' Health Protection in the Russian Federation shows the importance of decisions about the necessity and ways of providing medical care to dying patients, and the procedure is as follows: first, the physician makes a diagnosis and informs the patient (or his/her legal representative) about the best possible medical care for the particular patient in this particular situation; the patient (or his/her legal representative) makes his/her decision either to accept the doctor's advice or to act otherwise. However, it should also be noted that if the patient and his/her legal representative makes a decision that disagrees with the physician's opinion (i.e. evidence-based decision), the physician should explain the negative consequences of the decision.

Legislative norms regulating the procedure of obtaining informed consent and the confidentiality issue in special situations are reflected in several federal laws such as the Psychiatric Assistance and Rights of Patients (1992), On Transplantation of Human Organs and Tissues (1992), Blood and Blood Components Donation (1993), Prevention of Spreading of Disease Caused by Human Immunodeficiency Virus (HIV-Infection) in the Russian Federation (1995), Immunoprophylaxis of Infectious Diseases (1997), and other regulative documents regulating specific issues regarding medical or social assistance.

From the viewpoint of the ethical component in the legislation of the Russian Federation, such a key element as confidentiality of information obtained from the patient and about the patient in the course of his/her examination and treatment is worth mentioning. Confidentiality is guaranteed by the Law of the Fundamentals of the Citizens' Health Protection in the Russian Federation (Article 13) and the aforementioned Article 23 of the Russian Federation Constitution.

There are also general regulations that guarantee the protection of personal data contained in the Federal Law of Information, Information Technologies and Protection of Information 2006 and the Federal Law of Personal Data 2006.

Therefore, the Russian Federation legislation proclaims among the most important civil rights the right to life as the first fundamental natural right of Man, without which all other rights lose their meaning, because the dead do not need any rights (Matuzov 1998).

In the legislation of the Russian Federation there is no "right to die"; the state may only attest and legally certify death (in a special standard form — the death certificate), but has no right to allow or prohibit the person to die or kill oneself.

According to the law, homicide and incitement to suicide are crimes (Criminal Code of the Russian Federation, Articles 105 and 110). Besides, any attempt to assist a suicide, even if in mercy, may be considered only as an attenuating circumstance mitigating the punishment (Lebedev 2002). Besides, mercy killing (with or without the person's request) in medicine is prohibited in the Russian Federation (Article 45 of the Fundamentals). Therefore, currently, the law forbids euthanasia in Russia. Medical professionals are not allowed to perform euthanasia, i.e. to respond to the patient's request for hastened death by any actions (inactions) or any ways and means including the termination of life-sustaining treatment. The criminal law assumes that human life must be protected both during life and in the process of birth and death.

The definition of death has been described in Article 9 of the Federal Law of Transplantation of Human Organs and Tissues (1992); death is defined when brain activity ceases irreversibly (brain death), which is stated according to the procedure approved by the Ministry of Health of the Russian Federation.

Order No. 460, December 20, 2001, by the Russian Federation Ministry of Health approved the Guidelines for the Declaration of Death Based on Brain Criteria. In conformity with the Guidelines, the declaration of death implies a special procedure including the list of compulsory clinical criteria necessary for the declaration of brain death. Only after the protocol has certified brain death, may life-sustaining support be withdrawn.

Considering the ethical priority of the legal regulation of the medical futility issue in the development of the relevant section of the medical law in the Russian Federation, a number of international documents have been taken into account. Among those are the Nuremberg Code (1947), the Declaration of Helsinki (1964) with subsequent revisions and amendments, the Declaration of Alma-Ata (1978), the Declaration of Lisbon on the Rights of the Patient (1981), EC Recommendations for the EU Member States on the Organisation of Palliative Care (2003), the Belgrade Agreement (2005), the Declaration of Venice (2006), the Budapest Commitments at the EAPC Budapest Congress (2007), and the World Cancer Declaration (2008). These documents have largely contributed to the regulation of this issue in Russia.

In the case of providing care when treatment is considered futile, some international documents have been taken into account, such as the WHO guidelines on palliative care by the WHO Regional Office in Europe, the WHO Guidelines on the Palliative Care for Terminal Cancer Patients (2007), and the Joint Declaration and Statement of Commitment on Palliative Care and Pain Treatment as Human Rights (August 2008). It is because the importance of international cooperation is determined by the priority of international law established by the basic legal documents of the Russian Federation.

It should be mentioned that in regard to ethical issues concerning care at the end of life and futile medicine, provisions of professional codes in Russia are also important relevant guidelines. For example, the Physician's Oath is included in Article 60 of the Fundamentals, obliging physicians to be honest in performing their professional duty; to dedicate all their knowledge and strength to the treatment and prevention of diseases, and to the preservation and improvement of the health of people; to be always ready to provide medical care; to relate to the patient attentively and carefully, and to preserve medical confidences; to act in the patient's interests irrespective of the patient's religion, nationality, race, social standing or other circumstances; and to maintain the utmost respect for human life and never perform euthanasia.

According to the Medical Code of Ethics (at the Pirogov Medical Congress in July 1997), in providing medical assistance for a terminal patient, the physician must exert every effort to provide the necessary emergency care. The physician must not perform euthanasia or involve others in this practice, but he/she must relieve the sufferings of the dying patient by every available, known and permitted means. The decision about withdrawal of resuscitation, especially when there is no encephalographic evidence of irreversible brain death, should be made collectively where possible. The physician should respect the patient's right to spiritual support. The Ethical Code of the Russian Physician, approved at the Fourth Conference of the Russian Medical Association, in November 1994, gives a similar definition of the physician's conduct (Chapter 2, Article 14, "The Physician and the Patient's Right to Dignified Death").

Euthanasia as an act of deliberate termination of a patient's life, be it either at his/her request or at the request of the patient's family, is unacceptable; the same applies to passive euthanasia. Passive euthanasia implies the withholding of common treatment at the bedside of the dying patient. The physician must relieve the sufferings of the dying patient by all available and legal ways. Pain relief is absolutely essential (Novikov and Osipova 2005). The physician should guarantee the patient's right to spiritual support by a minister of any religious denomination.

FUTURE DEVELOPMENT ON THE ISSUE

In the twenty-first century, one of the key factors indicating the level of social civilization should certainly be the quality and availability of palliative medicine for terminal patients. The main principle of palliative care implies that each and every person has the right to receive medical care and be treated with equal dignity and respect in life and when facing death. As shown in this particular chapter, Russia has a long history of ethical and professional development of palliative medicine: in books, papers, manuals, laws/guidelines, medical, social, ethical and legal issues of end-of-life care are profoundly explored.

For further development of palliative medicine as well as dealing with medical futility in Russia, it is important to introduce palliative medicine as a specialty into the List of Medical Specialties of the Ministry of Health and Social Development. It is also crucial to stimulate further improvement of existing legislation, including new provisions on pain clinics, hospices, homecare teams, as well as setting standards for medical staff in palliative medicine, development of the federal system of statistical recording of patients who need palliative care, and development of protocols for disease management. Other important areas for future improvement in dealing with these issues include defining medical and economic standards for structure units, methodological principles with regard to the improvement of patients' quality of life with advanced chronic diseases. It could be helpful in future to encourage extra-budgetary funding (sponsorship from commercial and non-government public structures, religious institutions) to create new opportunities in this particular area.

To solve these issues, professional associations for palliative care specialists have been created to facilitate drawing out a unified national program for strategic planning of the palliative care development which has a close cooperation with the international society.

REFERENCES

Ekkert NV. 2006. Palliativnaja pomosch' // Organizacija i ocenka kachestva lechebno-profilakticheskoj pomoschi naseleniju // Uchebnoe posobie. — M., pp. 357–380.

Gnezdilov AV, Ivanjushkin AJa, and Millionschikova VV. 1994. Dom dlja zhizni (House for life), Chelovek, 5, pp. 116–121.

Ivanjushkin AJa and Hetagurova AK. 2003. Istorija i etika sestrinskogo dela. M., GOU VUNMC, p. 20.

Jubilee Bishops' Council of the Russian Orthodox Church. 2000. Bases of the Social Concept of the Russian Orthodox Church. Available at: http://orthodoxeurope.org/page/3/14.aspx.

Lebedev VM, ed. 2002. Kommentarij k Ugolovnomu kodeksu Rossijskoj Federacii. M., pp. 258–259 (Kommentarii k stat'jam 105, 110 — Krasikov Yu.A.).

Matuzov NI. Pravp na zhizn' v svete Rossiiskuh I mezhdunarisnyh standartov. "Provovedinije", 1998, No. 1, p. 198.

Modnikov OP, Rodionov VV, and Novikov GA. 2004. Kostnye metastazy raka molochnoj zhelezy (patogenez, klinika, diagnostika i lechenie). — M., Fond "Palliativnaja medicina i reabilitacija bol'nyh".

Novikov GA and Osipova NA, eds. 2004. Lechenie hronicheskoj boli onkologicheskogo geneza, M.

Novikov GA, Osipova NA, Rudoj SV, Prohorov BM, Vajsman MA, and Konstantinova MM. 2000. Palliativnaja pomosch' onkologicheskim bol'nym. Posobie dlja vrachej (recommendation for physicians). — M.

Novikov GA, Sokolov VV, Kabisov RK *et al.* 2001. Fizicheskie faktory v palliativnoj pomoschi onkologicheskim bol'nym. Posobie dlja vrachej (recommendation for physicians). — M.: Tipografija RIIS FIAN.

Novikov GA, Chissov VI, and Osipova NA, eds. 2002–2003. Problemy palliativnoj pomoschi v onkologii. Antologija nauchnyh publikacij. (anthologie of scientifique publication), — M., 3 volumes — Fond "Palliativnaja medicina i reabilitacija bol'nyh".

Novikov GA, Sokolov VV, Kabisov RK, Vajsman MA, Prohorov BM, and Rudoj SV. 2003. Metody korrekcii narushenij gomeostaza v palliativnoj pomoschi onkologicheskim bol'nym. Posobie dlja vrachej. — M., Tipografija Rossel'hozakademii.

Novikov GA, Akademika RAMN, Chissov VI, and Modnikov OP. 2004a. "Kurs lekcij po palliativnoj pomoschi onkologicheskim bol'nym" v dvuh tomah, M.

Novikov GA, Solov'ev VI, and Prohorov BM. 2004b. Palliativnaja pomosch' onkologicheskim bol'nym na regional'nom urovne. — Smolensk, FGUP "Smolenskaja gorodskaja tipografija".

Novikov GA, Chissov VI, Prohorov BM i dr. Sostojanie i perspektivy razvitija palliativnoj pomoschi onkologicheskim bol'nym. Kurs lekcij po palliativnoj pomoschi onkologicheskim bol'nym. V 2 tomah. T.1. — M., 2004c, p. 320.

Novikov GA, Prohorov BM, Vajsman MA, and Rudoj SV. 2005a. Kratkoe klinicheskoe rukovodstvo po palliativnoj pomoschi pri VICh/SPIDe. — M.: "Globus".

Novikov GA, Osipova NA, Prohorov BM, Vajsman MA, and Rudoj SV. 2005b. Palliativnaja pomosch' onkologicheskim bol'nym. Uchebnoe posobie (recommendation for education). — M., OOD "Medicina za kachestvo zhizni".

Novikov GA, Akademika RAMN, and Chissov VI, eds. 2006a. Palliativnaja pomosch' onkologicheskim bol'nym, M.

Novikov GA, Osipova NA, Prohorov BM, Vajsman MA, and Rudoj SVM. 2006b. Lechenie hronicheskoj boli onkologicheskogo geneza. Uchebnoe posobie. OOD "Medicina za kachestvo zhizni".

Silujanova IV. 2001. Etika vrachevanija: sovremennaja medicina I pravosla-vie. — M., pp. 246–247.

Zil'ber AP. 1998. Etika i zakon v medicine kriticheskih sostojanij. — Petrozavodsk, Izd-vo PGU, p. 560.

Zil'ber AP. 2000. Komfortnyj podderzhivajuwij uhod pri umiranii (eticheskie i juridicheskie aspekty). M.: Biomedicinskaja etika pp. 154–168.

CHAPTER SIX

MEDICAL FUTILITY IN AUSTRALIA

Dominique Martin

SUMMARY

This chapter reviews some of the recent literature concerned with end-of-life issues in Australia in order to provide an overview of the role of medical futility in end-of-life care in this country. It reveals an evolving approach to these issues that is influenced by a number of different domains of care, from general practice to intensive care units, and by a broad variety of decision makers governed by relatively new legislation and policy that concerns the use of advance directives.

Despite the absence of a formal definition of medical futility in Australian policies, a broad consensus on the key elements of the concept and the role they play in guiding ethical practice is evident both in the law and in professional guidelines. This is evident in policies governing resuscitation orders and in recent efforts to facilitate a legal framework for advance care directives and to promote the use of such directives. Australia is striving to achieve a better understanding of end-of-life care within society and the healthcare community, as well as to promote best practice in decision making about medical futility and end-of-life care.

INTRODUCTION

Most Australians enjoy the privilege of ready access to an excellent standard of healthcare and the benefits of recent developments in medical science. The average life expectancies of Australian men (79 years) and
women (84 years) are among the highest in the world. The relative abun-
dance of quality healthcare available to Australians comes at a significant
financial cost — 9.4% of GDP is spent annually on healthcare (AIHW
2011) — and also poses particular challenges for those involved in making decisions about care at the end of life. For as many as 50% of
Australians who die each year, death may be anticipated (Palliative Care
Australia 2005, p. 9), enabling patients and care providers to plan end-
of-life care and to make important decisions about such care. Despite the
wealth of treatments available, patients inevitably approach the limits of
contemporary medicine, where the failure of organ systems that precedes
death — regardless of the disease process or injury involved — can no
longer be reversed or stalled. At this stage, curative treatment is no longer
effective although palliative treatment, which aims to ease suffering rather
than halt or reverse illness, often remains useful. In some cases, although
treatment may be able to temporarily suspend the progression of disease
or compensate for organ failure, its failure to reverse the process and
achieve better health means that it is deemed effectively useless. In these
settings, further treatment aimed at restoring or preserving bodily functions may be deemed futile and the decision is made to withhold or
withdraw such treatment.

At a conceptual level, the definition of medical futility appears seduc-
tively simple. An intervention or treatment may be deemed "medically
futile" with respect to a particular goal that can be either specific and
quantifiable, such as the restoration of a physiological function, or more
complex and qualitative, such as the achievement of a patient's personal
health goals. The administration of adrenaline in the setting of cardiopulmonary resuscitation (CPR) might temporarily restore a cardiac rhythm,
but may not result in the patient's longer-term survival and discharge from
hospital. When making decisions about the utility of any treatment, medical practitioners and other decision makers must weigh the probabilities of
benefits and harms to the patient in the context of the patient's own preferences and goals. As far as possible, medical practitioners try to inform and

guide treatment decisions based on the best available evidence. Unfortunately, medicine remains an inexact science. Even where well-known treatments for common conditions are concerned, uncertainty remains.

Over large populations being treated, small risk probabilities mean that a few will nevertheless suffer rather than benefit from treatments. Where numbers suggest low probabilities of benefit, a lucky few may nevertheless make "miraculous" recoveries. Accordingly, making judgments about medically futile treatments in practice is fraught with difficulty, and especially so at the end of life, when the fear of giving up too soon may impair our ability to achieve a good death.

In the past decade, efforts to improve care at the end of life in Australia have resulted in new legislation, policies and guidelines, as well as numerous studies exploring current practices and attitudes to end-of-life care, and a growing body of literature that reviews and debates the issues raised in end-of-life decision making. Although medical futility is not always referenced in this work, it remains a core component of this field of study and practice. Providing end-of-life care entails at least a partial recognition that some forms of care are futile. This recognition enables decision makers and care givers to set aside treatments that may be unduly burdensome on patients, costly for healthcare budgets and distressing for families and care givers, and to provide palliative care. Importantly, recognition of medical futility with respect to a particular kind of treatment does not mean that all other forms of treatment are futile, or "merely" palliative. Distinguishing the role of palliative care in the setting of decisions about medical futility is a key issue in the Australian healthcare system.

THE HEALTHCARE SYSTEM IN AUSTRALIA

The Australian healthcare system consists of a national public healthcare program named Medicare. Funded by taxpayers, this program provides free emergency healthcare to all resident citizens and permanent residents (and visitors from other countries with reciprocity agreements) as well as healthcare for non-emergent conditions. It entitles those with Medicare cards to free treatment in public hospitals and from medical practitioners who "bulk bill", and to free or subsidized treatment by doctors, some dentists and optometrists for specified conditions. The public hospital system is jointly funded by state and federal governments and is administered at the level of state and territory governments. The system includes the Pharmaceutical Benefits Scheme (PBS), which provides essential medicines to all citizens, with copayments for those who do not have a Healthcare card — a welfare program that entitles them to free medicines. Under the Medicare system, most Australian citizens have access to an excellent level of care. On the other hand, waiting lists for non-urgent surgery, to see specialists and even to see general practitioners providing free care at "bulk-billing" clinics (which do not charge a copayment) may be painfully long. Furthermore, public patients have no freedom of choice of specialist. There is thus a thriving private healthcare system as well, which offers those who pay for private health insurance access to a range of services including private hospitals, specialists of choice and much faster access to non-urgent care. The government encourages participation in private insurance by penalizing those earning over a certain income who do not take out such insurance.

Costs and Decision Making in Australia's Healthcare System

Decisions to limit the essential medical care of an individual patient in Australia, regardless of whether they are privately insured or not, are never made on the basis of costs alone. Although a patient might exhaust the number of "free" allied health consultations they are offered by their insurer or the public system each year, or a work cover insurance company may refuse to fund a particularly expensive operation that the insurer deems is unnecessary or not related to the workplace injury, if a treatment is covered by Medicare, or a medication included in the PBS, these are unlikely — if ever — to be withheld simply on the basis of costs for a particular individual. Nevertheless, rising healthcare costs are an important concern for the government, with 121.4 billion AUD spent on healthcare in the year 2009–2010 (AIHW 2011). Consequently, healthcare providers are encouraged to minimize costs by avoiding unnecessary procedures, investigations and treatments and by the judicious provision of cost-effective care.

Futile care at all stages of life may include admissions to intensive care, surgical procedures, specialist medications, blood transfusions or simply prolonged hospital admissions that can produce enormous financial costs as well as directly impair access for other patients to receive such care who would be more likely to derive a benefit. These considerations undoubtedly influence practitioners in busy public hospitals who constantly face the pressure of increasing demands on finite resources — most obviously in the form of limited bed numbers.

Although the Australian government influences medical decision making through the regulation of funding and the creation of guidelines and policies governing particular practices such as organ donation and allocation, most decisions about medical care take place at a more individual level, in association with the patients concerned. Healthcare in Australia may be provided within a variety of domains, and deaths occur in various settings: 16% of Australians die at home, 20% in hospices, 10% in nursing homes and the rest in hospitals (Department of Health and Ageing 2011). Those involved in providing end-of-life care may be drawn from community care settings involving general practitioners, nurses or outpatient programs. Nursing homes, hospices and palliative care programs in particular may offer or facilitate the discussion of end-of-life issues. Within hospitals, the emergency department (ED), inpatient wards and the intensive care unit (ICU) represent three different domains of decision making. Movement between these areas or consideration of patient transfer between them may necessitate decision making about end-of-life care and the possible futility of various treatments.

Whether in the context of a possible admission to the ICU or a routine visit to a general practitioner, decision making about end-of-life care usually involves patients, their families and doctors. The advantages of community-based decision making often include a more relaxed and less time-pressured environment, familiarity between healthcare providers and patients and the ability of patients to participate. In hospitals, patients may be too unwell to participate in decision making, providers are likely to be unknown and unfamiliar with patient preferences, and decisions may need to be made within very short time frames under highly stressful conditions. On the other hand, the pressured environment of emergency and intensive care medicine may offer some advantages. Patients and their relatives may be more willing to confront the challenges of decision making when the prospect of death and the suffering associated with some conditions and treatments become a tangible reality. Furthermore, doctors required to act as "gatekeepers" to the ICU and those practicing emergency medicine may be better equipped and more accustomed to informing patients about the probabilities of treatment success, and the advantages and disadvantages of particular forms of care. End-of-life decision making and care in Australia may take place in many different settings, but the issues and challenges faced by patients and care providers are essentially the same regardless of the healthcare domain in which they occur.

Ethics and Issues at the End-of-Life

Ethical discussions about end-of-life issues in Australia, like those in many countries, are often framed by the principles of beneficence, nonmaleficence and respect for autonomy and human dignity. The multicultural nature of Australian society means that ethics in practice often requires sensitivity to and respect for a variety of religious and cultural values and practices that may influence the attitudes of patients and their families, as well as those of doctors, to the way end-of-life issues are understood, explored and expressed (e.g. Sneesby *et al.* 2011).

Respect for patient autonomy acknowledges the right of individuals to participate in decision making regarding their medical care. Competent patients are entitled to refuse treatment — even where it is thought to be life saving — and may in some cases choose between different treatment options offered by their doctors. However, patient autonomy does not entail a right to insist upon treatment that medical practitioners deem futile or harmful. Australian patients (or their proxy decision makers) who are dissatisfied with the options presented by their doctors may seek a second opinion, but cannot insist upon treatment where this has been refused by a care provider on the grounds that it is not in the patient's best interests. While medical practitioners are required to inform patients about treatment options and to consider patient preferences, facilitating their participation in decision making, respect for autonomy should never outweigh professional obligations to avoid harm and to promote the well-being of patients.

The individualized conception of autonomy that has dominated medical ethics for some decades has recently begun to evolve, as accounts of shared decision making and relational autonomy gain wider recognition. In Australia, cultural, ethnic, educational and linguistic barriers to communication and understanding between patients and care providers may compromise efforts to respect patient values and hence autonomy and to involve patients in decision making, especially about end-of-life care (Smith *et al.* 2009; Johnstone and Kanitsaki 2009). Inclusion of family members in decision making is a routine practice, although rarely driven by formal protocols. Documentation of not-for-resuscitation (NFR) orders, for example, usually has a place to note whether the family or next of kin has been involved in the discussion, but consultation with family is not mandated.

As patients approach the end of their lives, treatments tend to offer less therapeutic benefit and their potential side effects accordingly may appear disproportionately harmful. Many patients endure prolonged and frequent hospital admissions during their last year of life (Rosenwax *et al.* 2011), and may grow weary of intravenous cannulations and other "minor" invasive procedures, even where these offer therapeutic benefit. On the other hand, patients desperate to survive may demand extraordinary interventions in the hope of gaining more time or obtaining a cure, despite substantial evidence that such procedures may be harmful and will not succeed. It is the physician's role, in association with the patient and/or his/her family, to consider the potential therapies available and their advantages and disadvantages, in the light of the patient's evolving clinical condition and preferences. However, end-of-life care is often associated with significant costs to the Australian community, in particular through hospital admissions and emergency services calls (Kardamanidis *et al.* 2007). Where these costs are unnecessary and avoidable, they may compromise efforts to provide care elsewhere in the healthcare system, especially in the setting of limited resources. Thus recognition of futile care is essential in the ICU setting, for example, to ensure that access to the ICU is equitable. Australia's ageing population may place ever higher burdens on end-of-life care and will require careful management to ensure that healthcare is equitably distributed between all members of the community. Another important concern for justice in end-of-life care is that of equitable access to care, with some communities lacking adequate resources for palliative care and end-of-life care planning. In particular, remote indigenous communities may face significant access barriers to end-of-life care (McGrath *et al.* 2006).

In end-of-life care, the aim of care providers, patients and their families is to achieve "a good death". In essence, a good death involves minimal suffering, occurs at a time that cannot be significantly postponed and takes place in an environment conducive to the patient's well-being — perhaps at home, or in hospital, and in the presence of loved ones. To achieve this, in addition to providing standard medical care, respecting autonomy and promoting beneficence and avoiding harms, medical practitioners must be attuned to the spiritual, emotional and cultural needs of their patients and their family members, recognizing that good end-of-life care extends beyond the provision of standard medical care to include palliative care in its broadest conception. A further critical element for physicians is the ability to provide leadership in decision making which concerns the cessation or withdrawal of treatment, especially where treatment is identified as futile (see Murphy 2008). "Dying with dignity" is a popular phrase in Australian society and within the medical community. The concept of "dying with dignity" refers to both the minimization of suffering at the end of life, and the respect of patients' wishes and values in decision making.

The Australian Medical Association (AMA) in its 2004 Code of Ethics offers the following advice regarding care of the dying patient:

"1.4 The Dying Patient:

a. Remember the obligation to preserve life, but, where death is deemed to be imminent and where curative or life-prolonging treatment appears to be futile, try to ensure that death occurs with dignity and comfort.
b. Respect the patient's autonomy regarding the management of their medical condition including the refusal of treatment.
c. Respect the right of a severely and terminally ill patient to receive treatment for pain and suffering, even when such therapy may shorten a patient's life.
d. Recognise the need for physical, psychological, emotional, and spiritual support for the patient, the family and other carers not only during the life of the patient, but also after their death (AMA 2006a)."

MEDICAL FUTILITY IN AUSTRALIA: CONCEPTION, GUIDELINES AND REGULATIONS

At a basic conceptual level, an action is perceived to be futile when it fails to achieve a particular goal or goals. It is judged futile *with respect to* that goal or goals. Pre-emptive judgments regarding medical futility involve probability estimates of achieving benefits, just as do any medical treatment decisions. The longstanding international debate regarding definitions of futility arises from attempts to nominate specific goals or probabilities of success with which to identify futility, as well as from controversy regarding the role of futility assessments in medical decision making. Examining definitions of futility through the prism of CPR is helpful in clarifying the issues at stake.

The most simple conception of medical futility is that of a treatment that will not achieve the intended physiological effect in a particular case. Treatment success may be defined in a number of ways. The most basic goal of CPR is to restore the vital physiological functions which are suspended in cardiac or respiratory arrest. Immediately, time becomes another measure of success — how long will the heart or lungs continue to function after CPR is ceased? For example, cardiac rhythm and circulation may be restored for a few seconds during CPR, but this hardly qualifies as successful CPR. Furthermore, it surely could not be described as a benefit — however small — to the patient, as he is likely to be unaware of the transient restoration of his cardiac function. A minimal length of survival time is required to define successful CPR, but with increasing time other factors beyond mere restoration of circulation or breathing become involved. A patient may survive the arrest but be completely dependent on the continuation of other measures such as mechanical ventilation or intravenous infusions of cardiac drugs — both available only in the intensive care unit. Such an outcome is often described as a mere prolongation of death. However, although at a physiological level CPR has effectively only suspended the dying process, it may represent a benefit to the patient — if his family has the opportunity to see him before death, for example. Both physiological and personal or social goals thus become entwined. A physiological goal — for example, the possibility of surviving to particular milestones such as "breathing independently", or "being able to walk to the bathroom" — represents a benefit only with respect to the patient's preferences. Such goals may be easily quantifiable — for example, "length of survival time during which patient is able to breathe independently" — by physicians, but their qualitative value is less readily assessed.

The task of estimating probabilities of success is even harder than that of defining goals. Our pursuit of evidence-based medicine encourages patients and practitioners to think in terms of certain outcomes, yet we forget that even regularly prescribed medications offer only statistically probable benefits rather than guaranteed effects. Decision making at the end of life cannot hope to achieve any greater certainty than that which occurs throughout the spectrum of medical care.

No formal definition of medical futility exists in Australian legislation. Australian law recognizes a broad conception of futility that is both quantitative and qualitative. Willmott *et al.* (2011) suggest that Australian case law demonstrates provision of care must be in the patient's best interests, and that futile care by definition is not in the patient's interests. Further, that care which is unnecessarily burdensome or intrusive may also not be in the patient's best interests, and may thus be refused on those grounds. The idea of promoting best interests and avoiding harm points to a qualitative assessment of treatment goals, although this clearly retains a wide scope for definition of futility in practice.

Australian guidelines also sidestep the issue of quantifying probabilities of success and defining specific goals. The Australian Medical Association published a position statement in 2007 that offers ethical guidance for medical practitioners involved in care at the end of life. It confidently defines futility as follows:

"Futile treatment — Treatment is futile when it is no longer providing a benefit to a patient, or the burdens of providing the treatment outweigh the benefits" (AMA 2007).

It also presents a qualitative understanding of futility that highlights not only the role of patient preferences and values but also the idea of best interests of the patient as understood by medical professionals involved in care:

"10.2 Medical practitioners are not obliged to give, nor patients to accept, futile or burdensome treatments or those treatments that will not offer a reasonable hope of benefit or enhance quality of life" (AMA 2006).

As levels of certainty regarding physiological effects decrease, consideration of qualitative factors are likely to increase. Futility is a rationale essentially based on identification of specific goals which are considered to be of such value that, if their achievement is unlikely or impossible, no other benefits are to be considered in decision making. So (allowing for a qualitative interpretation of futility), if told there is no chance of my surviving discharge from the ICU following cardiac arrest and CPR, I may decide that CPR would be futile. I value that goal — being sufficiently well to survive independently of the ICU — so highly that *regardless of any other considerations* — including other potential benefits, for example giving my son time to say farewell — if it is not achievable, I decide not to have CPR. Thus estimation of futility is more than a calculation of possible advantages and disadvantages; it occurs prior to further decisions regarding the appropriateness of a particular treatment. If I decide it is not futile, I must then consider other benefits and whether I am willing to risk harms, and so on.

In end-of-life decision making, the choice of benefit(s) by which to measure the futility of a treatment is highly significant; if achieving this particular goal is unlikely or impossible, death is the preferred alternative. Use of the futility rationale thus highlights the extraordinary nature of decision making in end-of-life care. Not only does it emphasize that such decisions are more than mere cost-benefit calculations, it signals the need to explore the complexities of the deliberating process, and to acknowledge the qualitative and individual nature of value preferences involved therein.

Advance Care Directives

Although lacking the right to demand futile treatment, Australian common law dictates that competent individuals have the right to *refuse* treatment, whether beneficial or not. That is, the right to bodily integrity prevents forcible treatment where a patient is deemed competent to refuse. In the case of end-of-life care, where patients are often unable to consent or refuse treatment, efforts have been made to give patients a role in decision making through the use of advance directives. An advance care directive (ACD) is a document which outlines a patient's treatment preferences. Official designation of a medical enduring power of attorney (MEPA) may also form part of an ACD or an alternative to it, where a patient designates an individual to make decisions on their behalf in the event of them being incompetent to do so in the future. ACDs enable patients to prospectively play a role in decision making in their own end-of-life care, even where they are no longer competent to do so. Although not wholly concerned with futility, advance directives may effectively express patient judgments about futile treatments. For example, advance directives may refuse life-sustaining treatments in the event of the patient suffering severe dementia. This suggests that while treatment would successfully prolong life, it would fail to achieve the patient's qualitative life goals. ACDs often embody subtext regarding qualitative goals and the futility of pursuing treatment in the face of failure to restore or to achieve a certain quality of life.

The AMA endorses the use of ACDs as follows:

> "8.2 The AMA strongly promotes advance care planning as a process of supporting patient self-determination, including the development of advance directives and the identification of surrogate decision-makers such as Enduring Powers of Attorney (EPA) (or similar), as a means to ensure that the patient's values and goals of care are known. ACPs are prepared by the competent patient to assist in decision-making if he/she loses the capacity to make treatment decisions in the future (AMA 2007)."

Not all Australian jurisdictions have legislation recognizing the use of ACDs; however, "anticipatory refusals of treatment" are recognized in common law, "whether spoken or written" if five criteria are met:

> "(1) The person must have been competent when he or she formulated the advance directive.
> (2) The refusal of consent must have been made voluntarily, unequivocally, and without duress.
> (3) The refusal of treatment must represent a 'firm and settled commitment' rather than an offhand remark that informally expresses a reaction.

(4) The advance decision must have been made with reference to and intended to cover the particular circumstances which subsequently occurred.

(5) The person must have known in broad terms the nature and effect of the treatment to which he or she was refusing consent (Jordens *et al.* 2005)."

A 2009 survey of Australian intensive care doctors revealed variable responses to the use of ACDs in hypothetical scenarios, with a number of doctors acting in conflict with the advance care plan or the wishes of a medical enduring power of attorney (Corke *et al.* 2009). The authors suggest that lack of understanding of the legal status of such directives, as well as "personal differences in ethics, beliefs and responsibility" may result in variable decision making despite the availability of ACDs (p. 125). Another study of Australian emergency physicians found low rates of education regarding ACDs despite significant support for their systematic introduction and standardization in practice (Wong *et al.* 2011). The study demonstrated a clear influence of ACDs on treatment decision making among emergency clinicians, although consideration of the patients' conditions and comorbidities, as well as ethical concerns remained highly influential. It seems ACDs are an important and useful factor in decision making, but do not act as an outright replacement for the professional duty to consider and act in the patient's best interests.

Unfortunately, ACD ownership within Australia remains an exceptional practice. A 2003 study at a major tertiary hospital in Melbourne found that only 7.9% of patients entering the emergency department had some kind of ACD, although 82.6% expressed support for some form of ACD and 59.6% "had spoken with at least one person about how much treatment they wanted in the event of serious illness" (Taylor *et al.* 2003, p. 589). A more recent regional survey of aged care facilities in New South Wales found that the median prevalence of ownership of ACDs among residents was 5% (Bezzina 2009). Recent research is helping to identify the factors which must be addressed if ACDs are to play an effective role in end-of-life care in Australia. Numerous legal barriers to the implementation of ACDs are reviewed by Seal (2010), who advocates a national approach that would facilitate education and promote consistency in practice. Boddy *et al.*

(2012) review the challenges for medical practitioners striving to formulate and implement ACDs with patients, and authors such as Jeong *et al.* (2010) and Watts (2011) discuss the role of nursing staff in contributing to advance care planning.

Not-For-Resuscitation (NFR) Orders

A common element of many advance care directives is a not-for-resuscitation order, also known as a DNR or do-not-resuscitate order. Frequently, however, such orders are established during hospital admissions, and are generally intended to be reviewed if the patient's condition changes during admission, or at least on subsequent hospital presentations. Most NFR orders are distinct from ACDs in that they are developed in the acute setting, in the light of the patient's current condition and comorbidities, rather than in anticipation of a future state of affairs. Although originally designed specifically to preclude attempts to perform CPR in the event of cardiac or respiratory arrest, their scope has now widened to effectively constitute a more comprehensive care plan akin to ACDs within the hospital setting. They may include limitations on the use of inotropes, antibiotics, parenteral feeding or admission to intensive care. They may also be used to preclude initiation of medical emergency team (MET) calls, where a team urgently attends patients whose condition has suddenly deteriorated on the ward, with a view to implementing more intensive treatment and preventing progression to cardiac or pulmonary arrest. Typical NFR forms enable those completing them to indicate "yes" or "no" with respect to each form of treatment listed, including the use of palliative treatments. This helps to ensure that the medical needs of patients identified as being "NFR" are not simply ignored. Despite being identified as "NFR", a patient may well receive considerable benefit from treatments such as noninvasive ventilation or antibiotics. Patients for whom treatment has become purely palliative also require ongoing care that risks being ignored if hospital staff interpret "NFR" as being "not for any treatment", a danger that has been confirmed in some international studies (e.g. Smith and Bunch O'Neill 2008; Beach and Morrison 2002; Chen *et al.* 2008). Recent research in Australia and New Zealand suggested that "general medical patients admitted to hospital and documented as NFR carry a higher mortality risk and a prolonged LOS [length of stay] both of which are only partly explained by these patients' greater age and comorbidity" (McNeill *et al.* 2012, p. 68).

In a study in 2007 among Australian hospitals, 54% of surveyed hospitals had formal NFR policies, with 45% of these providing a "standardized order form" to document NFR orders, and 52% simply writing the order in patient notes (Sidhu *et al.* 2007, p. 73). Only 68% stipulated that the rationale for the order must be documented. Most contained space to document whether the order had been discussed with the patient and family (p. 75). Although "futility" is often invoked as a rationale for withholding CPR in the event of an in-hospital arrest, the degree to which such decisions are made using the best available evidence regarding the patient's condition, as well as the extent to which the patient's qualitative goals are considered is uncertain at best. Micallef *et al.* (2011) demonstrated strong levels of agreement on NFR order decisions among hospital specialists in Australia, suggesting that there is a reasonably consistent approach to decision making from the medical perspective. However, the same study also concluded that considerable barriers exist to timely decision making and documentation of NFR status, with the result that some patients suffer inappropriate resuscitation attempts. Shanmuganathan *et al.* (2011) offer suggestions for early identification of patients who may need their resuscitation status clarified prior to clinical deterioration.

MAKING DECISIONS ABOUT FUTILE TREATMENT: HOW AND BY WHOM

By now, it should be evident that decision making in end-of-life care in Australia is a complex process. Decision making may take place in a variety of settings, from aged care facilities to general practice clinics and emergency departments and intensive care units. For many Australians, it seems that decision making begins within the home, where discussion of treatment preferences in the event of serious illness may take place with family members (Taylor *et al.* 2003). The gradual evolution of advance care planning means that more formal decision making may involve patients, relatives, lawyers, and medical and nursing staff in the community or within healthcare institutions. At this stage, however, it seems probable that many decisions in Australia take place in the acute setting within hospitals, when a patient's condition deteriorates significantly or during the end stages of a terminal condition.

Depending on the clinical circumstances, in particular the severity of a patient's condition, the patient's capacity to participate in decision making and the extent to which the patient's death has been, or may be anticipated, decisions about the futility of particular interventions and the approach to further care may be made in a number of ways. In some cases, protocols may exist to guide and govern the structure of decision-making procedures whether in the formulation and documentation of advance care directives or NFR orders, or simply to facilitate a standard procedural approach from professionals involved. Usually, medical practitioners familiar with the patient's medical history and current condition review the patient's prognosis in the light of available treatments, often in consultation with specialists. Synthesizing this information, medical staff present the patient and/or their next of kin with a summary of the possible treatments and the likely benefits and risks of each. Often, patients are then able to express their own preferences, concerns about options and to identify personal goals they may have. Nursing staff may also be consulted and can play a key role in communicating patient preferences (Watts 2011). In some cases, patients will be advised of only a very limited range of treatments, which may simply be palliative. Presenting options such as surgery or more intensive care as futile, doctors will explain why these treatments are not an option. On the other hand, where the risks and benefits of potential treatments are equivocal, patients may be urged to make a decision between conservative or invasive treatment, with little definitive guidance from doctors. Some patients prefer not to play a role in decision making, delegating this task to their doctors or family members. In the case of pediatric patients, parents in Australia play a key role in decisions to withdraw or limit treatment at the end of life (Moore *et al.* 2008). Where agreement is not achieved between medical staff, patients and their families, pathways to resolution may be implemented, such as consultation or review by other medical staff, the involvement of patient advocates or hospital ethics board reviews. Rarely, the law becomes involved.

As we have seen, a variety of potential decision makers may be involved to a greater or lesser extent in end-of-life care. Formal surrogate decision makers for patients may have medical enduring power of attorney or guardianship. Parents act for their (minor) children, while in the case of incompetent patients with no surrogate, close family members are usually accorded decision-making powers. All parties involved in decision making are expected to act in the best interests of the patient. However, conflicts between healthcare providers and patients and their relatives most commonly arise through failure to communicate relevant information, to explain decisions and to consider and respect the preferences and values of the patient with respect to end-of-life care (see e.g. Forbes *et al.* 2008; Smith *et al.* 2009). Conflict can arise when patients (or their families) disagree with doctors regarding the futility of treatment, but perhaps just as frequently occurs when doctors continue to pursue treatment that patients or their families feel is overly burdensome and futile. In the latter case, however, it may be harder for patients to express their preferences, particularly to medical staff who may presume that most patients will prefer "active treatment". Nursing staff that spend more time with patients may be more receptive to the expression of preferences regarding the withdrawal of treatment, and may advocate on behalf of patients.

The Issue of Unilateralism in Decision Making

A frequent concern about the invocation of "futility" in medical decision making is that it may be used by doctors to make inappropriate and unilateral decisions that wrongfully deny patients life-saving care. Involvement of patients and their next of kin in decision making plays a key role in preventing misunderstandings and ensuring that patients' interests are promoted. In some cases, however, patients and/or their relatives or surrogate decision makers may disagree with doctors about the futility of a particular treatment. In situations of disagreement, a second opinion may be sought. Rarely, a care provider and/or a hospital may be sued by the patient or their surrogate. In such settings, Australian common law clearly upholds the right of doctors to refuse to provide or continue futile treatment that is not in the patient's best interests, regardless of family preferences. However, if the determination of futility is judged erroneous, medical practitioners are required by law to continue treatment (see Stewart 2011). On the other hand, the state of Queensland requires doctors to obtain consent for the withdrawal or withholding of treatment, even where such treatment is futile (Willmott *et al.* 2011). This creates a confusing situation in which, as Willmott *et al.* (2011) note, doctors may be legally required to act in violation of their ethical and professional duties by providing, at least temporarily, care that is not in the best interests of their patient. According to Stewart (2011), however, rather than forcing doctors to provide care that conflicts with their professional duty to act as they judge best for the patient, this added procedural element of futility determination helps to protect the patient's interests and provides pathways for review that enable doctors as well as the patient and their relatives to have a say in the decision-making process. Nevertheless, Stewart concludes, "Those responsible for the patient's care should bear in mind the views expressed but ultimately they must decide what in clinical terms and within the resources available is best for their patient" (p. 160).

EUTHANASIA AND MEDICAL FUTILITY

Patients or their relatives may on occasion ask medical staff to assist them in dying, in order to end suffering. A Victorian study found that 59% of doctors who have treated terminally patients have received "requests to hasten death by withdrawing or withholding treatment" (Neil *et al.* 2007, p. 722). The issue of euthanasia has been the subject of passionate public and professional debate in Australia for more than a decade. "Euthanasia" literally means "a good death"; however, it is commonly understood to refer to the practice of deliberately hastening death in order to relieve suffering. Various categories of euthanasia have been defined. *Voluntary* euthanasia is performed with the consent of the person who chooses to die, and is sometimes distinguished from assisted suicide in which a person is enabled to end her own life. *Involuntary* euthanasia is performed against the wishes of the person and is usually considered to be synonymous with murder. *Non-voluntary* euthanasia, on the other hand, occurs when the person is not able to provide consent. Finally, euthanasia is sometimes distinguished as active or passive, where active refers to actions such as the administration of drugs intended to hasten death, and passive refers to the withdrawal of (or failure to initiate) life-sustaining or -prolonging treatments with the intention of hastening death. A number of excellent critiques of the confusing and often misleading terminology surrounding euthanasia exist. Some have even suggested we should avoid the term altogether (e.g. Kuiper *et al.* 2007). I adopt here the terms commonly found in the Australian media and literature.

Some authors have argued that "passive euthanasia" is a misnomer; however, Garrard and Wilkinson (2005, p. 65) argue that where treatment is withheld or withdrawn for the purpose of hastening death, where this is deemed to be in the patient's best interests and where the intention is not simply to remove overly burdensome treatment, this constitutes passive euthanasia. Interestingly, they also exclude cases where treatment is withdrawn or withheld on the grounds of futility, that is, "incapable of benefiting the patient" (p. 65). If futility is construed broadly and qualitatively, it is easy to conclude that nearly all possible cases of passive euthanasia will in fact be judged simply the withdrawal of futile treatment. If treatment is judged capable of benefiting the patient on more narrow physiological grounds, for example where parenteral hydration maintains renal function and thus prolongs life, then withdrawal of fluids for the purpose of hastening death would count as passive euthanasia.

Most references to euthanasia in the Australian literature tend to be concerned with active euthanasia. In Australia, recognition of medical futility and the decision to withdraw or to withhold treatment is rarely referred to as "euthanasia". As noted earlier, Australian law supports the practice of withdrawing or withholding treatment deemed futile or not in the best interests of patients. Nevertheless, a 2007 study by Neil *et al.* showed confusion among the medical community in the state of Victoria regarding the definition of euthanasia, and whether withdrawal or withholding of treatment with the intention of hastening death also constituted euthanasia.

In 1995, the Northern Territory of Australia passed the Rights of the Terminally Ill Act (Bartels and Otlowski 2010, p. 540), becoming the first jurisdiction in the world to legalize active voluntary euthanasia (AVE). The law entitled competent adults suffering from a terminal illness to receive assistance to kill themselves. Applications to undergo euthanasia required signatures from three doctors including a specialist, and a psychiatric review to ensure the decision was not the result of a treatable depression. Following the deaths of only four patients, the Act was over-turned by the Euthanasia Laws Act 1997 which invoked (for the first time) a constitutional right allowing the Federal Parliament to make laws for the Australian territories and to invalidate a territory law — which had never before been invoked (p. 540). Subsequently, most Australian states have witnessed unsuccessful efforts to introduce legislation permitting AVE. In addition, the Federal Parliament in 2005 criminalized "the provision of information on how to commit suicide" in response to efforts by Australia's most well-known euthanasia campaigner, Dr. Philip Nitschke, to advise patients on methods of peaceful suicide (p. 541).

A number of the so-called mercy killings, assisted suicides or euthana-sia cases have been prosecuted in Australian law, usually involving rela-tives of the deceased. Bartels and Otlowski (2010, pp. 531–532) note that only one case since 2000 has resulted in a custodial penalty, largely due to the fact that it was atypical of euthanasia cases. Debate about the intro-duction of AVE legislation in Australia is ongoing, thanks to euthanasia support groups, campaigners such as Dr. Nitschke, the Australian Greens Party and other politicians who continue to put forward bills on the sub-ject. Newspapers and television programs report on court cases and patients who have traveled abroad to undergo euthanasia (e.g. Button 2007). Surveys suggest a significant proportion of the Australian public supports some form of legalized euthanasia (e.g. Horin 2011) and as much as 53% of medical practitioners (Neil *et al.* 2007, p. 723). Surveys also show that a large proportion of Australian medical practitioners have been asked by patients to hasten death, and 35% admit to deliberately adminis-tering drugs with the intention of hastening death at the request of a patient (p. 723). More commonly, doctors frequently administer palliative treatments with the intention of relieving suffering, but in full knowledge that a secondary effect of such treatments will be to foreseeably hasten death. The doctrine of double effect holds that in these circumstances, administering treatment is not euthanasia, and the treating medical staff are not responsible as such for the patient's death. In some cases, pallia-tion may be regarded as a grey area designed to mask euthanasia in the absence of a legal right to perform euthanasia. On the other hand, the Australian states of Queensland, Western and South Australia have legislated to ensure that doctors may safely offer patients palliative care without fear of prosecution. For example, the Consent to Medical Treatment and Palliative Care Act 1995 of South Australia states:

17. The care of people who are dying

(1) A medical practitioner responsible for the treatment or care of a patient in the terminal phase of a terminal illness, or a person participating in the treatment or care of the patient under the medical practitioner's supervision, incurs no civil or criminal liability by administering medical treatment with the intention of relieving pain or distress:
    (a) with the consent of the patient or the patient's representative; and
    (b) in good faith and without negligence; and
    (c) in accordance with proper professional standards of palliative care....

This Act subsequently makes clear that euthanasia is not permitted:

"18. Saving provision

(1) This Act does not authorise the administration of medical treatment for the purpose of causing the death of the person to whom the treatment is administered.
(2) This Act does not authorise a person to assist the suicide of another (White *et al.* 2011, p. 489)."

CONCLUSION

The concept of futility in medical decision making has a long and varied history. Contemporary medical practitioners and societies, at least in the privileged environments of developed nations such as Australia, need no longer fear that the outcomes of disease or injury are to be determined solely by prayer, willpower or fate when the contents of the doctor's bag are exhausted. Instead, we face a far more complex situation, in which it seems that there is always something more that might be offered by medical science in the hope of promoting recovery, prolonging life or alleviating symptoms: another operation, a new combination of antibiotics, a novel therapy. Even where actual therapies are non-existent, hopes may be pinned on holding out long enough to receive treatments that remain merely speculative possibilities, such as some genetic modifications and stem cell transplants. In this context, amidst the "mythos of regeneration" in modern medicine, it is difficult simply to say, "There is nothing more that can be done." Doctors, other healthcare providers, patients and their friends and family are left to struggle through a wealth of sometimes patchy and inconclusive information in order to answer the fundamental question which remains: "Is there anything more that ought to be done?"

In Australia, as is the case elsewhere, questions regarding the utility or futility of providing particular treatments in particular cases are shaped by a variety of concerns. Although in individual cases, doctors begin by considering the particulars of the specific patient at hand, the nature of modern healthcare is such that broader concerns about the availability of resources within hospitals and within wider healthcare systems inevitably play a role in decision making. For policy makers, resource issues are necessarily a major consideration in determining not simply what ought to be done for patients in particular circumstances, but also what can realistically be done in the setting of resource constraints, in order to respect broader social goals of justice and equity that may be less obviously at stake in the setting of individual cases.

Although the practical and ethical goals and values involved in decision making about treatment at the end of life are essentially the same as those that guide decision making about the provision of healthcare in general, the stakes appear higher as death approaches. The human costs of withholding treatment deemed futile at the end of life include untimely death — an error that cannot be reversed. On the other hand, the costs of providing genuinely futile treatment may be high at a personal level — with prolongation of suffering — and burdensome for strained healthcare systems facing ageing populations and ever-greater costs.

End-of-life care, decision-making models and procedures for advance care planning are emerging priorities in Australian policy, legislation and medical practice. Issues such as euthanasia and the limitation of treatment at the end of life are important subjects of debate within Australian families as well as among the professional healthcare community. Although considerable research is still needed to determine how best to implement more effective end-of-life care and decision making, the variety of existing models and research into both public and professional values and attitudes suggests there is substantial agreement among the diverse Australian population regarding the pursuit of a good death for each of us.

REFERENCES

Australian Institute of Health and Welfare (AIHW). 2011. *Health Expenditure Australia 2009–10.* Health and welfare expenditure series No. 46. Cat. no. HWE 55. Canberra: AIHW. Available at: http://www.aihw.gov.au/ publication-detail/?id=10737420435 [Accessed March 1, 2012].

Australian Medical Association (AMA). 2006. Code of Ethics — 2004. Available at: http://ama.com.au/codeofethics [Accessed March 1, 2012].

Australian Medical Association (AMA). 2007. Position Statement on The Role of the Medical Practitioner in End of Life Care. Available at: http://ama.com.au/ node/2803 [Accessed March 1, 2012].

Bartels L and Otlowski M. 2010. A right to die? Euthanasia and the law in Australia. *Journal of Law and Medicine* 17: 532–555.

Beach MC and Morrison RS. 2002. The effect of do not resuscitate orders on physician decision-making. *Journal of American Geriatrics Society* 50: 2057–2061.

Bezzina A. 2009. Prevalence of advance care directives in aged care facilities of the Northern Illawarra. *Emergency Medicine Australia* 21: 379–385.

Boddy J, Chenoweth L, McLennan V, and Daly M. 2012. It's just too hard! Australian health care practitioner perspectives on barriers to advance care planning. *Australian Journal of Primary Health*, doi:10.1071/PY11070 [EPub ahead of print].

Button J. 2007. My name is Dr John Elliott and I'm about to die, with my head held high. *Sydney Morning Herald*, January 26. Available at: http://www.smh.com.au/news/ world/a-doctors-sad-farewell/2007/01/26/1169788692086.html?page=fullpage [Accessed March 1, 2012].

Chen JL, Sosnov J, Lessard D, and Goldberg RJ. 2008. Impact of do-not-resuscitation orders on quality of care performance measures in patients hospitalized with acute heart failure. *American Heart Journal* 156: 78–84.

Corke C, Milnes S, Orford N, Henry MJ, Foss C, and Porter D. 2009. The influence of medical enduring power of attorney and advance directives on decision-making by Australian intensive care doctors. *Critical Care and Resuscitation* 11: 122–128.

Department of Health and Ageing. 2011. The National Palliative Care Strategy — Supporting Australians to Live Well at the End of Life. Available at: http://www. health.gov.au/internet/publications/publishing.nsf/Content/ageing-npcs-2010-toc~ageing-npcs-2010-introduction [Accessed March 1, 2012].

Forbes T, Goeman E, Stark Z, Hynson J, and Forrester M. 2008. Discussing withdrawing and withholding of life, sustaining medical treatment in a tertiary paediatric hospital: A survey of clinician attitudes and practices. *Journal of Paediatrics and Child Health* 44: 392–398.

Garrard E and Wilkinson S. 2005. Passive euthanasia. *Journal of Medical Ethics* 31: 64–68.

Horin A. 2011. Euthanasia wins 75% support. *The Age*, January 6. Available at: http://www.theage.com.au/national/euthanasia-wins-75-support-20110105-19g8h.html [Accessed March 2, 2012].

Jeong SY, Higgins I, and McMillan M. 2010. The essentials of Advance Care Planning for end-of-life care for older people. *Journal of Clinical Nursing* 19: 389–397.

Johnstone MJ and Kanitsaki O. 2009. Ethics and advance care planning in a culturally diverse society. *Journal of Transcultural Nursing* 20: 405–416.

Jordens C, Little M, Kerridge I, and McPhee J. 2005. From advance directives to advance care planning: Current legal status, ethical rationales and a new research agenda. *Internal Medicine Journal* 35: 563–566.

Kardamanidis K, Lim K, Da Cunha C, Taylor LK, and Jorm LR. 2007. Hospital costs of older people in New South Wales in the last year of life. *Medical Journal of Australia* 187: 383–386.

Kuiper MA, Whetstine LM, Holmes JL *et al.* 2007. Euthanasia: A word no longer to be used or abused. *Intensive Care Medicine* 33: 549–550.

McGrath P, Patton MA, McGrath Z, Ogilvie K, Rayner R, and Holewa H. 2006. "It's very difficult to get respite out here at the moment": Australian findings on end-of-life care for indigenous people. *Health & Social Care in the Community* 14: 147–155.

McNeill D, Mohapatra B, Li JY *et al.* 2012. Quality of resuscitation orders in general medical patients. *QJM* 105: 63–68.

Micallef S, Skrifvars MB, and Parr MJ. 2011. Level of agreement on resuscitation decisions among hospital specialists and barriers to documenting do not attempt resuscitation (DNAR) orders in ward patients. *Resuscitation* 82: 815–818.

Moore P, Kerridge I, Gillis J, Jacobe S, and Isaacs D. 2008. Withdrawal and limitation of life-sustaining treatments in a paediatric intensive care unit and review of the literature. *Journal of Paediatrics and Child Health* 44: 404–408.

Murphy BF. 2008. What has happened to clinical leadership in futile care discussions? *Medical Journal of Australia* 188: 418–419.

Neil DA, Coady CA, Thompson J, and Kuhse H. 2007. End-of-life decisions in medical practice: A survey of doctors in Victoria (Australia). *Journal of Medical Ethics* 33: 721–725.

Palliative Care Australia. 2005. A guide to palliative care service development: A population based approach. Available at: www.palliativecare.org.au/Portals/46/resources/PalliativeCareServiceDevelopment.pdf [Accessed March 1, 2012].

Rosenwax LK, McNamara BA, Murray K, McCabe R, Aoun S, and Currow DC. 2011. Hospital and emergency department use in the last year of life: A baseline for future modifications to end-of-life care. *The Medical Journal of Australia* 194: 570–573.

Seal M. 2010. Health advance directives, policy and clinical practice: A perspective on the synergy of an effective advance care planning framework. *Australian Health Review* 34: 80–88.

Shanmuganathan N, Li JY, Yong TY, Hakendorf PH, Ben-Tovim DI, and Thompson CH. 2011. Resuscitation orders and their relevance to patients' clinical status and outcomes. *QJM* 104: 485–488.

Sidhu NS, Dunkley ME, and Egan MJ. 2007. "Not-for-resuscitation" orders in Australian public hospitals: Policies, standardised order forms and patient information leaflets. *Medical Journal of Australia* 186: 72–75.

Smith CB and Bunch O'Neill L. 2008. Do not resuscitate does not mean do not treat: How palliative care and other modalities can help facilitate communication about goals of care in advanced illness. *Mount Sinai Journal of Medicine: A Journal of Translational and Personalized Medicine* 75: 460–465.

Smith SK, Dixon A, Trevena L, Nutbeam D, and McCaffery KJ. 2009. Exploring patient involvement in healthcare decision making across different education and functional health literacy groups. *Social Science & Medicine* 69: 1805–1812.

Sneesby L, Satchell R, Good P, and Van der Riet P. 2011. Death and dying in Australia: Perceptions of a Sudanese community. *Journal of Advanced Nursing* 67: 2696–2702.

Stewart C. 2011. Law and cancer at the end of life: The problem of nomoigenic harms and the five desiderata of death law. *Public Health* 125: 905–918.

Taylor DM, Ugoni AM, Cameron PA, and McNeil JJ. 2003. Advance directives and emergency department patients: Ownership rates and perceptions of use. *Internal Medicine Journal* 33: 586–592.

Watts T. 2011. Initiating end-of-life care pathways: A discussion paper. *Journal of Advanced Nursing* 68: 2359–2370.

White BP, Willmott L, and Ashby M. 2011. Palliative care, double effect and the law in Australia. *Internal Medicine Journal* 41: 485–492.

Willmott L, White BP, Parker M, and Cartwright C. 2011. The legal role of medical professionals in decisions to withhold or withdraw life-sustaining treatment: Part 2 (Queensland). *Journal of Law and Medicine* 18: 523–544.

Wong RE, Weiland TJ, and Jelinek GA. 2011. Emergency clinicians' attitudes and decisions in patient scenarios involving advance directives. *Emergency Medicine Journal* 29: 720–724.

CHAPTER SEVEN

MEDICAL FUTILITY IN JAPAN

Yasuhiro Kadooka and Atsushi Asai

SUMMARY

Medical futility is a difficult issue to resolve and its concept is elusive. Unlike in Western countries, little research has been performed on this theme in Japan. However, the questions set forth by authors in this article indicate that many Japanese healthcare providers have already recognized the significance of this issue. Japan uses universal health insurance, which supports social justice and healthcare access for all. Japan has a rapidly aging population, and boasts the highest longevity in the world. Excessive attention to the goals of sustaining life without considering the patients' personal wishes is considered the main problem of Japanese end-of-life care (Macer 2005). It is supposed that medical futility is an immediate problem that must be addressed in Japan. In this chapter, we describe the healthcare system, end-of-life issues, decision-making, related laws and guidelines, as well as euthanasia in Japan. We also show the results of our empirical survey on medical futility.

THE HEALTHCARE SYSTEM IN JAPAN

Japan's population, which has been steadily decreasing since 2005, was about 127 million in 2009. Children (0–14 years), the working-age group (15–64 years), and elderly people (≥65 years) constituted 13.5%, 64.5%, and 22.1% of the total population, respectively. The population is expected to fall below 100 million by 2045 (Japanese National Institute of Population and Social Security Research 2006). The declining birth rate and rapidly aging population are serious social issues. In 2009, there were 176,471 medical facilities (174,315 beds) in Japan. There were 8,739 hospitals, most of which were private clinics. The average daily number of hospitalized patients was 1,308,219, and the average daily number of outpatients was 1,416,845 (Japanese Ministry of Internal Affairs and Communications 2011; Ministry of Health, Labor and Welfare 2010). These numbers are nearly unchanged from the previous year.

The average lifespan in Japan was 79.59 years for men and 86.44 years for women in 2009 (Japanese Ministry of Internal Affairs and Communications 2011). The population aging rate in 2008 was 22.1%. Although health conditions were extremely poor in Japan immediately after World War II, the country currently enjoys the highest life expectancy in the world and stands as the leader in the "health Olympics: the rankings of country life expectancies". One of the reasons for the country's remarkable health gains is the effectiveness of its healthcare system (Bezruchka et al. 2008). Japan has had universal health insurance coverage extending to all citizens since 1961. In 2001, 2.25% of 20–59 year olds were uninsured. Almost the entire Japanese population is covered by this system. Insured members pay 30% of medical expenses, but burdens on the elderly, children, and low-income individuals are lower. Patients can choose hospitals and doctors and request healthcare services according to their preference. Furthermore, there is an upper limit to the amount patients pay; patients can receive financial assistance if the amount claimed is too large. Thus, insured members can avail themselves of expensive treatments. Such a system ensures universal accessibility and allows for achievement of optimal health outcomes.

A fee-for-service system has been implemented for individual treatment services since 1958. National health expenditure consists of health insurance funds (about 49%), taxation (about 37%), and copayments (about 14%). The system is blamed for the large number of hospital beds and long hospitalization periods, frequent medical examinations, and expanded use of medical tests, resulting in an inefficient healthcare system, relatively high drug expenses, and overtreatment of the elderly (Ikegami and Campbell 1995; Idezuki 2008; Wang *et al.* 2010). During high-speed economic growth, managing health resources may not have been difficult. However, these factors synergized and contributed to rising medical expenses and structural problems (Idezuki 2008). A rise in the aging population and advances in medical technology, among other factors, have led to an increase in national health expenditure, which amounted to 34.8 trillion yen (about 424.4 billion USD, 1 USD = 82 yen) in 2010. To solve this problem, cost-containment measures were implemented, including introduction of a flat-fee payment system called diagnosis procedure combination (DPC), an increase in the payment rates for the elderly, and fee schedule revisions. While these measures failed to reduce total medical expenditure, they did achieve some results: the average length of hospital stay was significantly reduced, patients could obtain more medical information, and the quality of medical treatment and hospital management improved (Wang *et al.* 2010). A high rate of aging population, accompanied by a deterministic population decline in the future, will affect the maintenance of the universal health insurance system and result in a possible healthcare resource crunch.

According to the Organisation for Economic Co-operation and Development (OECD) Health Data 2008, the practicing physician density (per 1,000 population) was 2.15 and total health expenditure (percentage of gross domestic product) was 8.1%. The values of both indicators occupied lower positions compared to those of other member countries. Conversely, the average length of stay for acute care was 18.8 days, hospital bed density (per 1,000 population) was 13.8, psychiatric care bed density (per 1,000 population) was 2.7, acute care bed density (per 1,000 population) was 8.1, computerized tomography (CT) scanners per million population was 97.3, and the density of magnetic resonance imaging units (per 1,000 population) was 43.1. These numbers were the highest among OECD member countries.

Although dealing with medical futility and allocating scarce health resources are substantially different problems, the aforementioned issues with the Japanese healthcare system, including the rapidly aging population, appear to be associated with medical futility. Bagheri anticipated that medical futility would be an emerging issue in the near future and would hit the ethical and health policy debates in Japan. In 2006, he and his colleagues conducted a questionnaire-based survey directed at Japanese bioethics specialists (Bagheri *et al.* 2006). Almost 60% of respondents believed that medical futility was an especially relevant issue in Japanese healthcare and that aggressive treatment could be stopped on medical futility grounds in spite of the available financial support. They concluded that along with the ongoing reform of the medical system, health insurance policies, and an increasingly aging population, discussions about medical futility and the application of life-sustaining treatments for marginal benefit would find more importance in Japan. However, there have been few expert discussions and investigations on this theme since Bagheri's effort. Presently, many Japanese people recognize that medical cost inflation is a serious social concern, but this has not led to increased discussions on medical futility. Little has been known about what ordinary Japanese people understand about medical futility and further research is needed to clarify it.

ETHICS IN END-OF-LIFE SITUATIONS IN JAPAN

Statistics published by the Ministry of Health, Labor and Welfare (MHLW) indicate that the total number of deaths was 1,141,865 in 2009 and that 80% of these occurred at medical facilities. According to a public survey conducted by the MLHW in 2008, more than 80% of laypeople wished to undergo end-of-life care and die in medical institutions (Japanese Ministry of Health, Labor and Welfare 2010). In Japan, which is already on its way to becoming a super-aging society, end-of-life care is an important concern. In the public survey, more than 80% of laypeople and 90% of healthcare workers expressed concerns about end-of-life care. The survey also revealed that almost 85% of healthcare workers felt distress and anxiety regarding end-of-life care and that 33.9% of medical doctors and 48.2% of nurses encountered disagreements on decision-making with regard to end-of-life care.

Most Japanese deaths are caused by chronic lifestyle-related situations or debilitating disease. Malignant neoplasm, stroke, and cardiac attack are the three main causes, which accounted for 344,105, 180,745, and 122,350 deaths, respectively, in 2009 (Japanese Ministry of Health, Labor and Welfare 2010). In particular, malignant neoplasm deserves the utmost attention. The Cancer Control Act, which formed the basis for the Cancer Control Propulsion Program, was established in 2007. The goal of this program is to reduce cancer deaths, improve the quality of life (QOL) of cancer patients, and diffuse palliative care. In Japan, hospice care was begun in the 1970s, and expanded after legalization and introducing the hospice care reimbursement in 1990.

Despite this, the impact of this program has not been strong enough. A total of 195 facilities were registered and the number of beds totaled 3,830 in 2009 (Okishiro and Tsuneto 2010).

Japanese physicians are hesitant to forgo life-prolonging treatments for terminally ill patients. This tendency was revealed through empirical surveys that compared the attitudes of physicians from different countries by using vignettes (Slutsky and Hudson 2009; Yaguchi et al. 2005). In everyday clinical settings, end-of-life decisions have been largely left to individual doctors because an institutional system for dealing with controversial issues in a team context does not exist and very few hospitals in Japan have a system for clinical ethics consultation (Aita and Kai 2006). In the case of considering termination of life-prolonging treatments for terminally ill patients, many Japanese physicians confront legal barriers because of the lack of relevant legislation and guidelines that protect physicians, emotional barriers, as well as cultural barriers because of physicians' paternalism and the lack of a method for determining formerly competent patients' preferences (Aita et al. 2007). However, it turns out that laypeople do not have a preference for aggressive life-prolonging treatments. A public survey conducted by the Ministry of Health, Labor and Welfare (MLHW) in 2008 reported that 89%, 95.3%, and 96% of laypeople did not wish to continue life-prolonging treatments if faced with imminent death without hope of recovery, a persistent vegetative condition, or a cerebrovascular accident (CVA)/dementia, respectively (MLHW 2010). The survey also revealed that 24.6%, 16.9%, and 13.5% of laypeople desired life-prolonging treatments if their family members were faced with the same three situations, respectively.

In Japan, there are no rules or laws regarding surrogate decisions and advance directives. It is unclear whether the guardian of an adult is authorized to make medical decisions. In a previous report on a clinical ethics consultation, a consultant team received questions about end-of-life care for incompetent patients from not only healthcare workers, but also families of patients (Fukuyama *et al.* 2008). In Japan, living wills are not legally effective and are rare; <1% of people have some form of advance directive at the time of death (Macer 2005). However, this situation may be changing. In a public survey conducted by the MLHW in 2008, 61.9% of laypeople and almost 80% of healthcare workers supported a living will for refusal of life-prolonging measures in end-of-life situations (47.6% and about 70%, respectively, in 1998) (Japanese Ministry of Health, Labor and Welfare 2010). The Japan Society for Dying with Dignity, established in 1976, demands the right to withdraw or withhold life-sustaining treatments and calls for legislation of living wills. Members of the organization write the wills, and its membership has continued to increase, reaching about 125,000 in 2010 (almost 0.1% of the population).

In 2009, interest in issues surrounding brain death increased with the revision of the Organ Transplant Law, which was prompted by problems associated with a shortage of donor organs from brain-dead patients (only 83 brain-dead transplants in 10 years under the old law) and criticisms of transplant tourism. The revision appears to have succeeded and brain-dead transplants are becoming more frequent. During the course of the revision, a question about the definition of death was raised: is brain death equivalent to the final death of a person? It was reported that, socially, people were increasingly accepting the idea that brain death equates to final death. However, under the revised law, the interpretation that "brain death is legal death" only applies in the context of organ transplants from brain-dead donors. There are still many cases in Japan where life-prolonging treatments, including mechanical ventilation, continue to be performed on brain-dead patients until cardiac death is achieved.

Japanese views on the body or the dead body are rooted in the Shinto religion. In Shinto, which is based on animism, the body is not a mere substance, but also something precious connected to the two gods that gave birth to the country. Cardiac death is perceived as natural death and the time of a soul's separation from its body. The body of the deceased should be treated as a person. Although views on life and death will likely change with time, it is an intrinsic value to maintain life as long as the body is alive, regardless of the condition. This means that medical workers have a duty to make an all-out effort to save a person's life even if s/he is in an irreversibly comatose state (Asai *et al.* 2010).

Cases associated with police investigation into ventilator removal from end-of-life patients and the cultural background behind decision-making in healthcare have triggered life-prolonging treatments, which invoke futility. Both of these situations are discussed further.

MEDICAL FUTILITY: RELATED LEGISLATION AND GUIDELINES

While basic laws on medicine exist in Japan, the Japanese penal code has not been revised to incorporate drastic changes to end-of-life care resulting from technological advances in recent decades (Aita and Kai 2006). There are no practical laws or procedures for the issue of medical futility, such as the Texas Advance Directive Law in the United States. No universally accepted definitions for medical futility have existed in Japanese society to date. This has led to increased anxiety about legal issues among healthcare workers.

In the case of medical futility, whether to forgo a treatment that is considered futile is a major issue. Although there is no precedent in Japan, some representative cases of mechanical ventilator removal from end-of-life patients at Hokkaido Prefecture Haboro Hospital and Imizu City Hospital found the life-prolonging treatments to be "meaningless" or "non-beneficial", as reported in some newspapers. The former case involved a patient in his 90s who recovered spontaneous heartbeat (without breathing) after resuscitation following cardiopulmonary arrest. The attending physician removed the respirator after evaluating the patient's brain-dead condition and determined that there was minimal chance of recovery. The latter was a case of respirator withdrawal involving seven patients aged 50–90 years, all comatose with end-stage diseases, between 2000 and 2005. In both cases, police reports on the attending physicians were sent to the prosecutor's office. However, none of the physicians were charged because a direct connection between respirator removal and patient death could not be established. The turmoil over withdrawal of care possibly places an unnecessary burden on dying patients and their families, misleads the mass media and public, and troubles police and prosecutors. The lack of legal and medical frameworks in Japan and the traditional practice of family-oriented decision-making (decision to withdraw respirators was reportedly made without knowledge of the patients' wishes and preferences) were cited as reasons for police involvement (Aita and Kai 2006).

According to a public survey conducted by the MHLW in 2008, 38.7% of physicians and 37.8% of nurses expressed a need for detailed standards or definitions for end of life and forgoing life-prolonging treatments (Japanese Ministry of Health, Labor and Welfare 2010). Although new laws have not been enacted, some guidelines regarding the forgoing of life-sustaining treatments for end-of-life patients have been developed in recent years. Forgoing such treatments may gain acceptance and social consensus in the near future. Medical futility is one of the important reasons for developing these guidelines which support the professional judgment of futility and withdrawal of life-sustaining treatments from terminally ill patients, but they do not provide unilateral authorization to healthcare workers. Three representative sets of guidelines are presented here.

The Guidelines Regarding End-of-Life Care in Emergency Medicine, developed by the Japanese Association for Acute Medicine in 2007, holds that the continuation of treatments that do not benefit a patient and are not desired by anyone, including the patient's family, undermines the patient's dignity and inflicts more suffering on the patient. These guidelines present four concrete end-of-life situations:

1) irreversible failure of whole brain function;
2) reliance on an artificial device due to irreversible lethal organ failure in the absence of alternative treatments;
3) the patient is expected to die within a few days despite continuation of treatment;
4) a condition that, after aggressive treatments, turns out to be the terminal stage of a malignant or irreversible disease.

The guidelines state that life-prolonging treatments can be forgone in response to a patient's advance directive, patient family's acceptance, and the medical team's careful judgment based on the best interest of the patient, and that the medical team should comply with the family's preference if they wish to continue treatment (Japanese Association for Acute Medicine 2007).

The second set is the Guidelines for the Decision-Making Process in End-of-Life Care, developed by the MHLW in 2007. It states that the decision to withhold or withdraw treatments from end-of-life patients is governed by patient preference and careful judgment by medical staff based on medical validity and appropriateness. The guidelines also discuss a need to establish ethics committees (Japanese Ministry of Health, Labor and Welfare 2007).

The third set is the Guidelines for Professional Ethics, developed by the Japan Medical Association and revised in 2008. It states that aimless prolongation of life for patients who have no hope of recovery and face imminent death is meaningless and damages dignity, that the patient's quality of life should be valued more, and that forgoing such treatments should also be considered. These guidelines regard the end-of-life condition (impossibility of treatment and inevitable death) and a patient's prior wish to forgo treatment as important considerations (Japan Medical Association 2008).

FUTILE TREATMENT: HOW AND BY WHOM DECISIONS ARE MADE?

The societal and political environments surrounding the patient-physician relationship and the decision-making process have gradually changed in Japan. The reigning principle underlying medical ethics is currently transitioning from paternalism to respect for patient autonomy. Western concepts, such as patient autonomy and informed consent, have slowly spread and people are now becoming more and more conscious of their rights as patients (Bito et al. 2007; Ito et al. 2010). However, the cultural facets of Japanese healthcare and society and the collective responsibility for patient care are very different from those that exist in Western countries, where such theories and principles were initially formulated (Ito et al. 2010).

The sick may prefer to leave decisions up to others or use subtle linguistic expressions to convey their will. However, there is still a hierarchical social system, that makes it difficult for patients and doctors to be truly at par in their relationship. Many sick persons are afraid to be a bother or burden to others, so they attempt to avoid trouble that could occur if they clearly expressed their will and it differed from that of others (Macer 2005).

Japanese patient-physician relationships are said to have four underlying characteristics that differ from those in Western cultures: collectivism, Confucianism, masculinity, and high context (Ishikawa and Yamazaki 2005). With respect to collectivism, individuals are consistently conceptualized as a part of a larger group and are expected to subordinate their personal goals to those of the group. Confucianism, which views harmony and obedience as virtues, has an impact on hierarchical and paternalistic relationships and family relationships, which are stronger than in Western countries. In particular, family members are more actively involved in the patient-physician relationship, and decisions are made within this triadic relationship.

With the right to privacy guaranteed by the Constitution, confidentiality is commonly written in many professional ethics codes or laws for health-care workers, and the Personal Information Protection Law went into effect in 2005. However, there are common exceptions in clinical settings. In a public survey conducted by the MHLW in 2008, 77% of laypersons indicated that they knew about the poor curability of their disease. Nevertheless, in such cases, 8.7% of physicians indicated that they would inform the patient first (3.4% in 1998) and 33.6% indicated that they would inform the family before informing the patient (58.8% in 1998). Moreover, regarding decision-making in such situations, 18.5% of physicians responded that they would ask the patient for an opinion (8.5% in 1998) and 21.6% responded that they would ask the family (35.2% in 1998) (Japanese Ministry of Health, Labor and Welfare 2010). Another survey, which investigated the desired involvement in healthcare decision-making, revealed that both the patient and family members wanted the family's involvement in medical decision-making, and concluded that the family plays a crucial role in healthcare decision-making, even when patients are competent to make their own decisions (Ito *et al.* 2010). Japanese healthcare workers must take into account the psychological benefits of the family, which in some cases provides no quantitative or qualitative benefits to the patient in some cases.

A questionnaire survey conducted by Bagheri and colleagues in 2006 included many questions on decision-making regarding medical futility, in addition to its expected impact on the Japanese healthcare system (Bagheri *et al*. 2006). A majority of respondents believed that the refusal to offer or continue treatments on the grounds of a judgment of futility can never be morally justified, that futility of the treatment should be evaluated on the basis of the doctor's medical judgment and the patient's value judgment. They responded that the patient/family preference and consideration about available health resources are important factors for evaluating futility. The study indicated that physicians should not be empowered to impose evaluative judgments that conform to professional standards and social interest. They concluded that there was no support for a physician's unilateral decision-making about futile care and that respondents were in favor of shared decision-making. The findings of the survey were similar to arguments presented in North America (Jecker and Perlman 1992; Tonelli 2007). This survey, however, suffers from two limitations: the small sample size and the fact that respondents were bioethics expertise who may have been influenced by Western bioethics principles. Findings from this survey may not sufficiently reflect Japanese attitudes toward decision-making in futility cases.

ATTITUDES OF HEALTHCARE PROVIDERS AND THE PUBLIC ON MEDICAL FUTILITY

Like Bagheri *et al*., we also felt the need for empirical surveys to explore the futility issue. The underlying issue is a disagreement between patients and healthcare workers, particularly the physician, on forgoing a treatment that invokes futility. We have investigated the differences in attitudes between the two groups. To this end, we conducted a preliminary interview study directed at Japanese healthcare workers (Kadooka *et al*. 2011). Participants of the study presented many cases that had been judged futile and stated the reasons for providing such treatments. A summary of the cases that have been judged as futile treatment, factors in futility judgment, and reasons for providing such treatments are shown in Tables 1 to 3.

Table 1.   Summary of Futile Treatment Cases.

Patient disease state (number of patients)	Treatment provided
Debilitated by terminal cancer (8)	Chemotherapy/surgical procedure
Unlikely to survive due to severe postoperative complications (4)	All forms of life-saving treatment
Patients with persistent vegetative state due to suicide or cardiopulmonary resuscitation (3)	All forms of aggressive treatment
Brain-dead patients (3)	All forms of aggressive or life-saving treatment
Unlikely to survive due to multiple organ failure (3)	All forms of aggressive treatment
Neonates unlikely to survive due to severe chromosomal aberration (2)	All forms of aggressive treatment
Alcoholism with hepatic cirrhosis (1)	Repeated treatments for esophageal varices
Unlikely to survive due to severe head injury (1)	Craniotomy procedure
Acute myocardial infarction, unlikely to return to spontaneous circulation (1)	Coronary artery catheterization procedure
Common cold (1)	Antibiotic and intravenous hydration
Infertile patient guessed to be menopausal (1)	Fertility treatment
Repeated aspiration pneumonia combined with severe dementia (1)	Pneumonia treatment
Bedridden with advanced dementia, unable to take orally (1)	Endoscopic gastrostomy
State of shock, terminal stage of brain tumor (1)	Administration of vasopressor agent
Arrhythmia and severe dementia (1)	Pacemaker implantation
Incompetent elderly with cardiac disease with poor quality of life that cannot improve (1)	Cardiac surgery

Most cases involved aggressive or life-sustaining treatments for end-of-life patients or incompetent patients who had already lost their competency. Healthcare resources were not considered in the context of allocated funds, but rather a balance between cost and benefit. Reasons for providing such treatments included factors other than patient request. These results are consistent with the suggestion of Bagheri *et al.* in their study. Discussions

Table 2.   Factors for Judging Futility in the Cases.

1   Patient's physical condition

2   Objective medical information

3   Treatment effects

4   Treatment risks

5   Preferences on the part of the patient

6   QOL of the patient

7   Psychological burden on the part of the patient

8   Balance between costs and benefits

9   Societal norms

Table 3.   Reasons for Carrying Out Treatments Judged as Futile.

1 Request for treatment from the patient

2 No refusal of treatment by the patient

3 Inadequate decision-making process (patient's inadequate understanding, healthcare worker's inadequate explanation, awkwardness of discussing stopping treatment, time/effort needed to persuade patients)

4 Inadequate relationship between the healthcare worker and patient (no trust or acceptance on the part of the patient, neither side wants to experience unpleasant feelings)

5 Instruction to give treatment from other physicians (senior physician, attending physician, primary care physician)

6 Feeling of guilt toward the patient (due to treatment complications)

7 No standards for judging futility

8 No standards, education, or regulations on forgoing treatments

9 Societal understanding that refusing requests from the patient is not allowed

10 Inadequate ideas and education about perspectives on life and death

11 The facility is a public institution

from a macroscopic perspective may also be required to resolve this issue. Subsequently, we designed a questionnaire survey based on the results of our initial study. The survey targeted not only Japanese healthcare workers but also laypeople, and attempted to evaluate differences in attitude toward medical futility in the two groups. The survey is likely to suggest that the attitudes of the two groups are different and that this issue pervades Japanese clinical settings. Quantitative data analysis is underway and the results will be published in the near future.

THE LINK BETWEEN MEDICAL FUTILITY AND EUTHANASIA

Past empirical surveys have shown that some Japanese healthcare workers actually carried out active euthanasia (Asai *et al.* 2001; Morita *et al.* 2002). However, euthanasia is not permitted by Japanese law. Penal Code Article 202 prohibits assisted suicide and homicide with consent. Two cases of active (non-voluntary) euthanasia received considerable public attention in Japan. In both cases, attending physicians were convicted of homicide. In the Kawasaki Kyodo Hospital case trial, an irreversibly comatose patient died after removing the ventilator and administration of muscle relaxant at the request of the patient's family. In this case the Yokohama district court (first trial) discussed the legality of forgoing life-prolonging treatment for end-of-life patients with respect to two necessary conditions: the patient's right of self-determination and the limits of treatment obligation. The latter rationale referred to medical futility:

> "If the physician provided appropriate treatments and the effectiveness reached its limit, there would be no legal obligation for physicians to continue or provide treatments judged as being medically meaningless, despite the patient's wishes. In such case, it could be said that the physician would not have a legal obligation to provide treatment and that forgoing treatment would be permissible."

According to the verdict, the physician's value judgment regarding the patient's death was inappropriate and physician judgment should have been limited to treatment effectiveness.

However, the higher court (the second trial) pointed out four problems with this rationale:

First, it is not clear at what point (probability of survival) the treatment was deemed meaningless, and second, the rationale does not override the physician's obligation to continue treatments as long as the probability of survival exists. Third, there are no considerations for the principle that the physician's best efforts until patient death is a mere call for professional ethics, and finally, it is presumed that forgoing life-prolonging treatments according to this rationale is an omission. Although a necessity for social deliberation on this rationale was argued, there has been no progress on arguments about its validity. The rationale has not achieved adequate social consensus for forgoing futile treatments.

CONCLUSION

In Japan, the main trigger for considering medical futility, which has not yet been studied and argued adequately, appears not to be the avoidance of conflicts between healthcare workers and patients. As Bagheri *et al.* pointed out, the issue has emerged along with an ongoing reform of the healthcare system and end-of-life care. The healthcare system has reached an equitable level and almost no one is prevented from seeking medical care for economic reasons. Under such circumstances, Japanese healthcare workers can provide meticulous or thorough treatments to some extent. Our recent study will be likely to present differences in attitudes between healthcare workers and laypeople toward medical futility. The determination of medical futility is based on moral judgments about treatment appropriateness at the bedside. The treatment goals and benefits, which include the patient's value judgments, must be identified before considering futility. While futility judgments may be diverse in each case, what drives patients to undergo treatments that are considered futile by healthcare workers? Empirical surveys as well as arguments based on theoretical assumptions are also important in resolving the remaining issues in Japan.

Many Japanese healthcare workers probably encounter futility in clinical practice given their professional or value judgments. It can be difficult for Japanese healthcare workers to insist on futility and refuse such treatments in disadvantageous situations, such as a lack of insufficient arguments, lack of specific laws regarding end-of-life care, and precedence for police involvement. However, it should be noted that the patient's family's excessive involvement in decision-making makes it difficult to identify the net benefit to the patient and leads to implementation of futile treatments. Good communication and relationships between healthcare workers and patients and their families will help avoid the futility issue to some extent. Guidelines or laws regarding medical futility, which may gain public consensus, are also desirable not only for the relief of healthcare workers, but also for the fulfillment of the patient's best interest and provision of appropriate treatments.

REFERENCES

Aita K and Kai I. 2006. Withdrawal of care in Japan. *The Lancet* 368: 12–14.

Aita K, Takahashi M, Miyata H, Kai I, and Finucane TE. 2007. Physicians' attitudes about artificial feeding in older patients with severe cognitive impairment in Japan: A qualitative study. *BMC Geriatrics* 7, doi:10.1186/1471-2318-7-22.

Asai A, Kadooka Y, and Aizawa K. 2010. Arguments against promoting organ transplants from brain-dead donors, and view of contemporary Japanese on life and death. *Bioethics* 26: 215–223.

Asai A, Ohnishi M, Nagata SK, Tanida N, and Yamazaki Y. 2001. Doctors' and nurses' attitudes towards and experience of voluntary euthanasia: Survey of members of the Japanese Association of Palliative Medicine. *Journal of Medical Ethics* 27: 324–330.

Bagheri A, Asai A, and Ida R. 2006. Experts' attitudes towards medical futility: An empirical survey from Japan. *BMC Medical Ethics* 7, doi:10.1186/1472-6939-7-8.

Bezruchka S, Namekata T, and Sistrom MG. 2008. Improving economic equality and health: The case of postwar Japan. *American Journal of Public Health* 98: 589–594.

Bito S, Matsumura S, Singer MK, Meredith LS, Fukuhara S, and Wenger NS. 2007. Acculturation and end-of-life decision making: Comparison of Japanese and Japanese-American focus groups. *Bioethics* 21: 251–262.

Macer D. 2005. End-of-life care in Japan. In: RB Blank and JC Merrick, eds. *End-of-Life Decision Making: A Cross-National Study.* Cambridge, MA: The MIT Press, pp. 109–129.

Fukuyama M, Asai A, Itai K, and Bito S. 2008. A report on small team clinical ethics consultation programmes in Japan. *Journal of Medical Ethics* 34: 858–862.

Idezuki Y. 2008. Long live the health care system in Japan. *Bioscience Trends* 2: 50–52.

Ikegami N and Campbell JC. 1995. Medical care in Japan. *New England Journal of Medicine* 333: 1295–1299.

Ishikawa H and Yamazaki Y. 2005. How applicable are western models of patient-physician relationship in Asia? Changing patient-physician relationship in contemporary Japan. *International Journal of Japanese Sociology* 14: 84–93.

Ito M, Tanida N, and Turale S. 2010. Perceptions of Japanese patients and their family about medical treatment decisions. *Nursing and Health Sciences* 12: 314–321.

Japanese Association for Acute Medicine. 2007. Available at: http://www.jaam. jp/html/info/info-20071116.pdf [Accessed April 2011] (in Japanese).

Japan Medical Association. 2008. Ishino-shokugyourinnrisisinn-kaiteiban (Guidelines for professional ethics). Available at: http://dl.med.or.jp/dl-med/ teireikaiken/20080910_1.pdf [Accessed April 2011] (in Japanese).

Japanese Ministry of Health, Labor and Welfare. 2007. Shumatsukiiryouno-ketteiprosesuni-kannsuru-gaidorain (Guidelines for the decision-making process in end-of-life care). Available at: http://www.mhlw.go.jp/ shingi/2007/05/dl/s0521-11a.pdf [Accessed April 2011] (in Japanese).

Japanese Ministry of Health, Labor and Welfare. 2010. Available at: http://www. mhlw.go.jp/stf/shingi/2r9852000000vj79-att/2r9852000000vkcw.pdf. Please see also; Japanese MHLW. 2010. Available at: http://www.e-stat.go.jp/SG1/ estat/List.do?lid=000001066473 [Accessed April 2011] (in Japanese).

Japanese Ministry of Internal Affairs and Communications, Statistics Bureau. Available at: http://www.stat.go.jp/data/nihon/02.htm [Accessed May 2011] (in Japanese).

Japanese National Institute of Population and Social Security Research. 2006. Available at: http://www.ipss.go.jp/shoshika/tokei/suikei07/suikei.html [Accessed April 2011] (in Japanese).

Jecker N and Perlman RA. 1992. Medical futility: Who decides? *Archives of Internal Medicine* 152: 1140–1144.

Kadooka Y, Asai A, Aizawa K, and Bito S. 2011. Japanese healthcare workers' attitudes towards administering futile treatments: A preliminary interview-based study. *Eubios Journal of Asian and International Bioethics* 21: 131–136.

Morita T, Akechi T, Sugawara Y, Chihara S, and Uchitomi Y. 2002. Practices and attitudes of Japanese oncologists and palliative care physicians concerning terminal sedation: A nationwide survey. *Journal of Clinical Oncology* 20: 758–764.

Okishiro N and Tsuneto S. 2010. Present situation and challenge of palliative care in Japan. *Nihon Rinsho* 68: 754–755 (in Japanese).

Slutsky A and Hudson LD. 2009. Care of an unresponsive patient with a poor prognosis. *New England Journal of Medicine* 360: 527–531.

Tonelli MR. 2007. What medical futility means to clinicians. *HEC Forum* 19: 83–93.

Yaguchi A, Truog RD, Curtis JR *et al.* 2005. International differences in end-of-life attitudes in the intensive care unit. *Archives of Internal Medicine* 165: 1970–1975.

Wang K, Li P, Cheng L, Kato K, Kobayashi M, and Yamaguchi K. 2010. Impact of the Japanese diagnosis procedure combination-based payment system in Japan. *Journal of Medical Systems* 34: 95–100.

CHAPTER EIGHT

MEDICAL FUTILITY IN CHINA: ETHICAL ISSUES AND POLICY

Yongxing Shi, Mingjie Zhao, Yang Yang, Cunfang Mao, Hui Zhu and Qingli Hu

SUMMARY

In China, due to the unique cultural background and economic conditions, terminal care ethics highlights as a "family culture". Based on the Chinese culture, the authors prefer to elaborate futile medical care and palliative care together under the issue of hospice care. By explaining the Chinese healthcare system, end-of-life ethics, relevant legislation and professional codes of hospice care, and the distinction and similarity between euthanasia and futile medicine, this paper presents a series of challenges in dealing with futile medical care in China.

The article suggests that only by providing education in end-of-life issues, improving the social security system, establishing multi-channel financing, adjusting the current medical insurance policy and integrating social volunteer teams, can the problems in dealing with medical futility be solved in China.

THE HEALTHCARE SYSTEM IN CHINA

Since the founding of the People's Republic of China, promoting people's health has been taken as the primary responsibility and an important mission by the Chinese government. In the healthcare system there are four main health policies; the first is the worker-peasant-soldier health policy, the second is preventive medicine, the third is the policy to combine traditional Chinese medicine with Western medicine and the fourth is the policy on integrating healthcare with mass movement.

The Labor Insurance Act instructs the state to provide preventive and medical care to all workers in the industry and mining sectors; to establish the Rural Cooperative Medical Care System; and to set up a urban-rural preventive healthcare network. All of these policies have contributed to the great improvement of the Chinese people's health status. The Constitution of the People's Republic of China states that "the state protects people's health... to develop social insurance, social assistance and medical care, all of which are required for the protection of citizens' rights."

Under the protection of the legal system, the Chinese government continues to improve the health management system and healthcare reforms, in order to provide advanced healthcare and better services to the people.

The average life expectancy of the Chinese population increased from 35 years before liberation (1949) to 73.5 years by the year 2011. In fact, China has improved the health status of one quarter of the world's population by only using 1% of the world's health expenditure (Ministry of Health 2009).

As mentioned, in China the issue of medical futility is dealt with under the issue of hospice care; however, compared to basic medical care, hospice care is less regulated which has a negative impact on futility decisions and patient referrals to hospice care. In today's China the annual new cancer cases are around 160 to 200 million, and there are more than 300 million existing cancer patients with an increasing trend of 3% per year. The number of deaths among cancer patients is about 1.4 million per year; however, the cancer cure rate is only 20%. Therefore, the application of futile medicine is becoming an emerging issue in the healthcare system in China.

Medical Insurance System in China

The healthcare system systematically subsidizes, allocates and applies health resources to improve the health of the population. It is an integral sector of the social security system and also a sign of a country's political system, economic and cultural progress, as well as social civilization (Cheng 2010).

In China, the healthcare system consists of the healthcare delivery system, medical insurance system and health surveillance system, all of which constitute a complete health system. In China, 90% of the health service institutions, located in both urban and rural areas, belong to three government administrative systems. One is the local government system at all levels (province, autonomous region, city and county levels), the second is the relevant state ministries and commissions system and the third is the Ministry of Health which includes the State Administration of Traditional Chinese Medicine. Due to the dual economic structure of the urban and rural areas in China, healthcare in urban and rural areas have a different evolutionary development history. The Basic Medical Insurance System is applied for urban residents, while the New Rural Cooperative Medical Care System is provided for rural residents.

The Chinese medical insurance system is composed of three types of supports: basic medical insurance for urban workers, basic medical insurance for urban residents and the New Rural Cooperative Medical Care System for rural residents. Meanwhile there are the medical aid system and commercial health insurance as supplements to the official insurance system, these including civil servants' supplementary insurance, enterprise supplementary medical insurance, and insurance for serious disease. These various types of healthcare systems are able to cover both the employed and unemployed population in urban areas, rural residents and the poor in both areas. Basic medical insurance for urban workers is provided to employees in state-owned enterprises, foreign-invested enterprises and joint ventures, with a drugs list for national basic medical insurance, injury insurance and maternity insurance. Basic social medical insurance for urban residents is provided to other urban residents, including the unemployed, the elderly, children and students at school, with the national essential drugs list. The New Rural Cooperative Medical Care System is provided to rural residents with its own drugs list. Commercial health insurance, social medical insurance and social medical aid complete the whole social medical insurance system. The medical aid system is provided to those swamped with unaffordable medical care.

Regarding the healthcare reimbursement policy in China, the three parties of the state, the collective and individuals proportionally share the reimbursement cost. The medical insurance fund is coordinated and managed by medical insurance agencies which are independent from the healthcare system, and are governed at all the different levels of the Administrative Bureaus of Human Resources and Social Security. Social medical insurance is one of the five fundamental aspects of social security. Basic medical insurance for urban workers is a major part of social medical insurance; its target population is the employee living in the city. This is a new type of social security system adapting to China's development at its primary stage of socialism. It should be noted that the medical insurance fund is centrally raised, managed and accommodated by the social medical insurance institutions; however, patients have to bear part of the medical costs based on their salary. The maximum amount of individual medical expenditure corresponds to their income; the rest would be covered by the mutual fund of medical insurance. The New Rural Cooperative Medical Care System is a peasant-mutual-aid system organized, governed and supported by the government, with the voluntary participation of farmers, which raises funds from individuals, units and state, based on the comprehensive arrangement for supporting patients with serious disease and mutual assistance and aid. The system has been designed in a way that the health insurance will give more compensation for in-patient services than out-patient, and more compensation for serious diseases than minor illnesses.

The Chinese medical insurance system provides free basic medical care for urban and rural residents; free basic public health services, such as residents' health records; healthcare management for children under six years old; management of maternal healthcare; elderly health management; hypertension disorder management; and patients with severe mental diseases etc. Currently, China covers the basic medical insurance of 1.2 billion people. There are 280 million insured urban employees across the country and 2,729 counties (cities, districts) have started the

New Rural Cooperative Medical Care System, with the participation of 924 million people.

It should be mentioned that the medical insurance payment system has an important impact on the decision-making regarding futile treatment and hospice services in China. For example, insured patients (in-patient or out-patient) can get reimbursement if they suffer from malignant tumors or impaired renal function, or require radiation therapy, chemotherapy, or long-term kidney dialysis. Therefore, in most medical conditions involving all those treatments, even if there was an issue of medical futility, as long as the patients were insured all the costs were covered.

So far, none of the Chinese social health insurance systems explained in this article has established any program to cover hospice care in the case of withdrawal of futile treatment. The vast majority of hospice services for terminal care are not included in their scope. Therefore, the lack of payment systems and policies in this regard affects the implementation of hospice care and futility decision seriously. This has caused problems in dealing with end-of-life issues in China.

ETHICAL ISSUES IN END-OF-LIFE CARE IN CHINA

The ethics of end-of-life care is an interdisciplinary subject, which applies general ethical principles in terminal care (Du and Hui 2003). The fundamental theory of ethics of end-of-life care, including deontology, the rights theory and professional ethics, is the most basic starting point in the ethics of end-of-life care.

At present, the ethical issues that need to be discussed in terminal care are fairness, autonomy and respect as well as sharing responsibilities. The principles of benevolence, autonomy, do-no-harm and respect of life are the foundations of the ethics of end-of-life care. The ethics of end-of-life care in China mainly focuses on the following topics: death and dying, rights of terminal patients, relationship between terminal patients and doctors, withdrawing treatment and excessive futile treatment, emergency care and rescue, social and religious supports, terminal patients and their families, ethical environment of terminal patients, terminal sedation, euthanasia, and hospice care.

In Chinese culture, death is something to be repelled and terrified of, and it is also a taboo to talk about death. The old saying of "a bad life is better than death" reflects the concept of death for a considerable number of people, who have no scientific education about death and dying. Therefore, when death comes, it is very difficult for patients and their families to accept it. In China, the issue of medical futility has been considered part of hospice care and palliative care dealing with patients at the terminal stage of their life. However, in dealing with terminal care patients, based on the traditional view, talking about the patient's death, palliative care or futile medical care is a taboo for the family members as well as the healthcare professionals. Based on the patient's medical condition, when treatment is considered futile, hospice care refers to providing appropriate medical care for the patient whose life expectancy is no more than six months in hospital or at home, aiming at alleviating his or her symptoms and slowing down the development of disease (Shi and Wang 2009, 2010).

In hospices, medical professionals control the symptoms of patients with their skills and good care rather than pursuing invasive, painful or meaningless treatment. Therefore, hospice care is bound to involve caring for a variety of symptoms in terminal cases, if providing aggressive treatment is futile. Palliative medicine as defined by the World Health Organization (WHO) is an approach that improves the quality of life of patients and their families facing the problem associated with life-threatening illness, through the prevention and relief of suffering by means of early identification and impeccable assessment and treatment of pain and other problems, physical, psychosocial and spiritual (WHO 2007). In China, physicians try to follow the WHO's practice and guidelines on palliative care, and as described by the Chinese words "宁养院" or "临终关怀病房", that is "hospice care hospital" or "hospice care ward", end-of-life care is provided in those centers.

In practice, a great challenge for terminal care is the traditional Chinese view of death, in which the end of life or death is inauspicious and the greatest "evil". The general attitudes towards death in China is "cherishing life but dreading death", so most of the irreversibly terminally ill patients are treated in the traditional way, with their meaningless lives prolonged by applying modern medical technology. Moreover, Chinese medical professionals always feel unprepared when faced with unconscious patients who are at the irreversible terminal stage of life, confronted with the moral dilemma of the traditional medical ethics core value of "retrieving the dying and rescuing the wounded."

There is no clear definition of the concept and the stage of end of life in China. Normally it refers to the elderly, patients with AIDS and patients with advanced cancer facing death in a very short time. Terminal care includes medical care for dying children, adults and the elderly in the terminal stage. Another understanding of the stage of end of life is the time process between life and death, which takes either a long or a short time. This is a necessary lead-time before the end of life, and consists of gradual changes in the quantity and quality of the patient's life.

The end-of-life stage can be divided into two categories: the reversible and the irreversible phases. The former refers to the stage of a disease, which is reversible by the application of modern medicine, although the patient's condition will deteriorate while the disease is worsening. The latter refers to the situation where the patient is undergoing an expected survival period in which modern medical measures can do nothing to save the life beyond its expected term. However, in some cases it is extremely difficult to make judgments about whether the patient's condition is in the reversible stage or the irreversible stage.

Withholding and Withdrawing Treatment

The concept of withdrawing treatment in a broader sense refers to terminating the ongoing treatment of curable and incurable patients due to various reasons. The narrow concept refers to the termination of a treatment that has no therapeutic value for the patient. Complete withdrawal means discontinuing all the treatment measures and letting the patient die; partial withdrawal means removing the main treatments but keeping the essential medication or the life support machine for the patient. Hospitals, physicians, patients and their families have their own reasoning and motivation for withdrawing treatment or requesting its continuation.

The current and general situation in China is that doctors in ICUs are aware when the patient is at the terminal stage and providing aggressive treatment has no meaningful result, and withdrawing the treatment and life support is a reasonable decision. However, the doctors will decide neither to withdraw nor to propose to the family to withdraw the patient's treatment; instead, they will sustain the treatment to the end, where an important measure of indication — the quality of life — is ignored. This explains why over-treatment is a relatively common practice and serious phenomenon in China.

As explained earlier, death in Chinese culture is considered a taboo and people do not talk about it, and a life of suffering is considered better than death. Therefore, in our view, death education is an urgent task, especially public education for the awareness of the concept of "a good death", as well as palliative and hospice care. Such a program should support the development of a better relationship between healthcare providers and patients and their family (Wang 1998).

Hospice and Palliative Care in China

In China, there is no consensus on the definition of medical futility, neither an explicit definition nor a clear explanation. So in practice it always relies on the descriptive explanation of symptoms, leading to the difficulty in defining related terms such as end of life, dying patients, terminal stage and its process, hospice care, technology and the ethics of terminal care. There are even difficulties in naming hospice agencies and their services, describing their functions, core values, professional responsibilities and service objectives (Shi 2010).

Hospice or palliative care is an emerging discipline of healthcare in China; however, there is no unified name for the agencies that provide terminal care. Most of the Chinese scholars suggest changing the term "terminal care" as it goes against the traditional Chinese culture. The medical professionals believe the term "end of life" increases the difficulty of communicating with patients and their families, and is especially sensitive, irritating and unacceptable for the elderly, and emotionally rejected by patients' families as well. However, as a medical term, "hospice care" has been used by the Ministry of Health, and by using terms such as "palliative care", people can make a connection with its real meaning.

The World Health Organization takes the accessibility of palliative care as a basic human right. The WHO made a practical definition of palliative care in 1990, the revision of which in 2002 states: "palliative care, as a worldwide urgent demand, should be taken as an important part of national health policies by every country". Although the goals of palliative care or hospice care are very clear, in China the health management system and traditional culture have not adequately adapted to this idea. Therefore, there is a lack of institutional and structural system to address patients' needs through the application of hospice care at the end of life.

The first terminal care research institution in China, the Hospice Care Research Center, was established on July 15, 1988, by a Chinese-American physician, Dr. Huang Tianzhong, and President of Tianjin Medical College Dr. Wu Xianzhong and Vice-president Dr. Cui Yitai at Tianjin Medical College. In March 1991, the First National Conference and Workshop of Hospice Care was held, after which five workshops on end-of-life care were carried out. In May 1992, the Ministry of Health decided to incorporate hospice care into the national health development plan.

Since 1990, the hospice agencies have developed in China with various structures: there is hospice care in general hospitals, specialty hospitals and community health service centers in some major cities. However, there are not so many hospice service centers in small cities and rural areas. According to statistics, in 2006 there were over 200 hospice care institutes in China, and in 2010 Shanghai with a population of 23 million had only three registered hospice care facilities. In Shanxi Province with 30,000 deaths from cancer annually, there were only two hospices. Until July 2011 only one hospice agency was established in Jiangxi Province. On February 25, 2010, the Standing Committee of Zhengzhou municipal government issued a regulation in its Suggestion on Accelerating the Development of the Pension Services of Zhengzhou City, requiring those hospitals that have the capacity to set up "hospice care wards or institutions". Since its initiation in 1998, the National Hospice Care Project has been supported financially by Mr. Li Ka-shing, a businessman from Hong Kong. This project set up 100 hospice care institutes in China, providing end-of-life and palliative care, especially for cancer patients, as "people-centered, holistic care."

Hospice care in China provides comprehensive palliative care for those patients in whom aggressive treatment is futile. In the program, a high-quality team addresses the patient's need through clinic visits, free home services, out-patient counseling and telephone follow-up. Providing services to poor people with respect to the patient and his or her family is their priority.

However, according to the Quality of Death Report by the Economist Intelligence Unit (EIU) of the Economist Group, which listed the quality of terminal care in 40 major economies, the highest ranked was the UK, followed by Australia, New Zealand and Ireland, while China ranked fourth from the bottom (EIU Report 2010).

POLICY DEVELOPMENT IN MEDICAL FUTILITY AND HOSPICE CARE

The health administrative departments have not developed regulations and professional codes for hospice care, nor set up any service policies, rules and regulations, and there were no technical standards or supervision and assessment programs. Therefore, there is a lack of professional codes and guidelines in dealing with futile medicine in hospice care.

Based on the regulation of social benefits, the right of terminal patients is a legal issue; however, there is no particular legislation to govern the issues related to terminal care patients in China. There are some related regulations such as the right of privacy and the right of confidentiality. Meanwhile, the rights of autonomy, informed consent, medical surveillance, partial exemption from social obligation, appeal and claim, as well as the right to die are well discussed in China.

Currently, there is no major support for hospices from the government and hospice care has not been a real priority for health resource allocation in China. At present, all of the hospice agencies with different names comply with the general health and medical regulations for medical institutions, which have been developed by the state and provinces. Under the planned economy system, their operations followed the policies of getting profits from drugs, charging the patients for all costs of medical examination and treatment. This kind of commission charge mechanism is based on the drive for profits. Therefore, this kind of service and behavior is far away from the WHO's concept of palliative care, and hospice care in China is still at the infant stage of its development.

In 2006, the Ministry of Health and the State Administration of Traditional Chinese Medicine issued the Notice of the Urban Community Health Service Management Measures (Trial) allowing hospice centers to be a conditionally registered health entity. The Notice for the first time expresses that hospice care can be registered as an independent department in a community healthcare center, providing a legal guarantee for terminal care in the community health service center, though there is still a lack of corresponding admission standards and regulations. Therefore, the terminal care service cannot be functional in the community healthcare services in a real sense.

In order to improve hospice care as an appropriate method to deal with medical futility, it should be integrated into the national social security system.

Currently, due to the lack of financial support, the existing hospice care institutes are unsustainable and find it difficult to run long-term. Therefore, it is necessary to develop supportive policies at the national level, to encourage multi-channel financing, and to establish a hospice care foundation. However, improving the volunteer organization system and expanding the volunteer teams would also be very important instruments.

DIFFERENCES AND RELATION BETWEEN EUTHANASIA AND MEDICAL FUTILITY IN CHINA

The Chinese term for euthanasia first appeared in AD 562–642, in the book *Collect of Peace and Happiness* by Dao Zhuo in the Tang Dynasty. It described peace and happiness as an alias for the Western Paradise where Buddhists would go after death. The original meaning of euthanasia in China is "in the spirit of a good end", based on the ideological foundation of the traditional culture.

The Chinese concept of euthanasia is defined in the Law Volume of the *Chinese Encyclopedia* as follows: "Under the sincere request of the dying patients with irreversible diseases who cannot be saved by modern medical technologies, doctors provide measures to end their lives earlier in order to reduce the unbearable great pain."

Therefore, euthanasia in China is defined as the process of dying patients who suffer from an incurable disease, because of the extreme mental and physical pain, being provided with humane medical intervention to end their lives without pain, which is requested by the patients themselves, their families and with the permission of the doctors. However, euthanasia is not widely accepted in China today due to the traditional view of death and the theory of the value of life. Chinese scholars believe that euthanasia is a kind of choice between dying in peace and dying in pain, and it is also a state and means of being in a good condition during the dying process (Du and Hui 2003).

Currently in China, neither the Chinese cultural and moral tradition, social status nor legislation system provides justification for euthanasia. In particular, the traditional Chinese culture shows that life is to be treasured and rejects death, which leads the majority of the public to reject euthanasia in the modern sense. At present, China has not passed any legislation on euthanasia; however, it is undergoing an attitude change from cautious opposition in the earlier debate to the current active advocating of euthanasia legislation by some social groups. The strict distinction between medical futility and euthanasia, as well as a rigorous procedure, is still being explored.

Several cases of euthanasia have happened since the 1980s, all of which were suicide with medication or other means with the assistance of the patients' families who could not bear to see the patients with incurable disease suffering in pain. However, all those involved have been prosecuted for their criminal liabilities.

Although active euthanasia is illegal in China, passive euthanasia has been practiced in many places. Research on the death of patients with critical care in some hospitals showed that 20% of the total deaths happened after passive euthanasia.

The Hanzhong Case in 1986 triggered a lively discussion of euthanasia, and it was the first case where the doctor was considered innocent of providing euthanasia.

In April 1987, during the conference of China's Sixth National People's Congress, Wang Qun and 31 representatives proposed Proposition 101, suggesting legislation for the Euthanasia Ordinance, which brought the issue of euthanasia legislation for the first time into the agenda for legislature. Since 1992, the National People's Congress has received proposals on euthanasia legislation annually, and in 1998, the research group led by

Zhu Shina of Shandong University of Traditional Chinese Medicine developed a draft proposal, "Provisional Regulations on Euthanasia". This was a significant progress and great achievement for euthanasia legislation. As mentioned earlier, although euthanasia is still a controversial issue in China, passive euthanasia has been practiced secretly and quietly in some cities such as Shanghai for a long time. However, the concept of euthanasia is not acceptable under Chinese law and medical institutions in China have not officially approved passive euthanasia.

In the case of futile medicine, palliative care is a special service given when there is no reasonable hope of cure and treatment does not provide any benefit, but may waste medical resources and do harm or even be against the dignity of patients. Such services include medical care, nursing, psychological and social care, which aim to control the symptoms, relieve the pains and promote the quality of life, and respect the life. It is comprehensive humane care for terminal patients (Wang and Li 2005). As Meng (2011) says, both euthanasia and hospice care in the case of futile medicine aim to make the dying process more comfortable and peaceful, and to relieve the pain and suffering. Both have the same goals of relieving the psychological and physical pain of terminal patients at the end of their lives. However, the concepts of euthanasia and medical futility have different origins, and there is a difference in the means of ending life and the attitudes toward death. Euthanasia emphasizes the dignity of death, but futile medical care or hospice care emphasizes the dignity of life; euthanasia focuses on the painless and fast death of terminal patients suffering from psychological and physical pain in a short process other than long-term care. However, providing hospice care when facing futile medicine involves comprehensive and long-term care for the patient's body, mind and spirit with appropriate and supportive care to the end. The implementation of euthanasia will leave a psychological shadow for patients' families, but hospice care will comfort them while facing medical futility.

A study done by the authors show that among 904 participants (physicians and nurses), 759 (83.98%) believe that euthanasia and medical futility are closely related; 316 (35.29%) of them think that the application of medical futility is in fact passive euthanasia. Only 56 (6.25%) participants said that these two are unrelated. If withdrawing futile medical care is considered euthanasia in a broader sense, and euthanasia is taken as the goal and procedure of dealing with futile medical care, the relation between euthanasia and medical futility should be harmoniously integrated. They should not be considered as contradictions but as similarities integrating with each other. Our idea is that all terminal patients should be provided with palliative care or a choice of euthanasia in the case of futile medicine, only by which hospice care in China can become ideal. In fact, only by integrating both, can the current public needs be met to the maximum extent and the brighter prospects of development be realized.

AN EMPIRICAL SURVEY ON ETHICAL ISSUES IN TERMINAL CARE IN CHINA

In order to provide some empirical data in this chapter about medical futility in China, and to get a deeper insight into the attitude towards terminal care in general and medical futility in particular, a quick survey was conducted from November to December in 2011. A questionnaire was sent to 950 healthcare providers in 66 medical and healthcare institutions, using stratified quota random sampling, in eight cities in different provinces. These were the municipalities of Beijing, Shanghai, Kunming, Guangzhou, Chengdu, Changchun, Ningbo and Huzhou. In principle, 30 participants from each general hospital and nursing home were selected, comprising 15 physicians and 15 nurses; and 10 participants from each community healthcare center, with five physicians and five nurses. In total, 904 responses were received, the response rate was 95.15%, and the statistical analysis was done using SPSS 12.0. The questions were designed to gather some demographic data and to cover five aspects of terminal care — terminal care ethics and policies, social response to terminal care, medical futility, hospice care and euthanasia — with 12 categories and 40 entries in total. A qualitative analysis method was employed and the data was loaded to Epi-data 3.02, and consistency checking and logical correction was conducted on the data.

Among the participants, 448 (49.61%) were physicians, 439 (48.57%) were registered nurses and 17 (1.82%) participants were social workers.

Of the 904 participants who responded with their view on legislation and policy regarding terminal care, 822 (90.36%) said that the Ministry of Health should stipulate regulation on terminal care, and 741 (81.25%)

respondents thought that the state government should adopt legislation on terminal care. Of them, 732 participants believed that a professional standard and code of conduct should be developed for dealing with medical futility. Of them, 813 (90.63%) participants considered that providing terminal care respects life and 85.16% of them believed that the principles of beneficence, autonomy, non-maleficence and respect for life were the main ones in providing terminal care. Among the 904 participants, 759 (83.98%) thought that euthanasia and medical futility were closely related; 316 (35.29%) thought that the application of medical futility was in fact passive euthanasia; only 56 (6.25%) participants said that these two were unrelated.

Comparing the results from different hospitals in this survey, we see that the respondents' opinions regarding the relation between euthanasia and medical futility are unevenly distributed based on different cities, occupations, education levels, ages and working experiences. Of them, 479 (53.26%) responded that in the case of medical futility, a joint decision by doctors and the patient's family was necessary and 475 (46.09%) of the participants believed that the patients should have the right to make their own decision. However, 198 (21.6%) thought that family members should make the decision and only 51 (5.6%) believed that physicians could make a unilateral decision regarding futile medicine.

In this study, participants from various professions shared the same view that in the case of medical futility physician and family members should make a joint decision. When asked about disclosure of a terminal diagnosis or changes in the patient's condition, and who should be notified first, 735 (81.38%) of participants believed that the patient's family should be notified first; 126 (13.93%) participants chose the legal representative and only 37 (4.04%) participants thought that the patient should be informed first. Regarding withdrawal of life-sustaining treatment, 630 (69.66%) participants believed that family members should be consulted first, 406 (44.92%) believed that physicians should communicate this with the patients, and 142 (15.76%) thought that physicians should tell the patients directly; only 39 participants said that they preferred not to talk about it with their patients. When asked for their views on whether patients with late-stage malignant tumors should be encouraged to accept the futility decision and the option of palliative care, 742 (82.03%)

responded that they would encourage patients to accept the decision. However, 102 (11.33%) participants expressed that they would not encourage patients to do so, and the remaining 60 (6.64%) participants responded that they would consult with their patients.

Regarding advance directives, 366 (40.49%) said that none of their patients had an advance directive and 437 (48.31%) participants had very few patients with advance directives.

CONCLUSION

In China, due to the unique cultural background and economic conditions, terminal care ethics is highlights as a "family culture". Therefore, based on the Chinese cultural influence on this issue the authors prefer to discuss medical futility as part of palliative and hospice care. In this article, to explore the concept of futile medicine, the Chinese healthcare system, the ethics of end-of-life care, related legislation and professional codes as well as euthanasia have been discussed. The paper pointed out a series of problems in dealing with futile medical care in China.

The results of the empirical survey presented in this chapter showed that the respondents believed it was necessary to have a legislation to govern end-of-life issues in general as well as medical futility in particular. The majority of respondents believed that the ethics of terminal care was mainly an issue of respect for human dignity and the value of life. Regarding the decision-making authority, they expressed that decisions about futile medicine should be a shared decision made by both physician and the patient's family. The majority (82.63%) said that they would encourage their patients with advanced malignancy to accept the futility decision and receive hospice care. This survey clearly indicates that healthcare professionals expect the Ministry of Health to develop relevant guidelines and policies about medical futility.

The paper suggests that providing public and professional education about death and dying, improving the social security system, supporting multi-channel financing, reforming the current medical insurance policy and integrating social volunteer teams are crucial in the better management of end-of-life issues in China.

REFERENCES

Cheng X. 2010. *Medical Insurance*. Shanghai: Fudan University Press, pp. 261, 282, 296.

Du Z and Hui E. 2003. *Medical Ethics Dictionary*. Zhengzhou: Zhengzhou University Press.

Economist Intelligence Unit Report. 2010. The quality of death ranking end-of-life care across the world. Available at: http://www.eiu.com/site_info. asp?info_name=quality of death_lien foundation&page= [last visited Dec 20, 2012].

Meng J. 2011. Discussing the harmony and unity of euthanasia and hospice care. *The Chinese Health Service Management* 3: 204–206.

Ministry of Health of the People's Republic of China. 2009. *Chinese Health Statistics Yearbook 2009*. Peking: Peking Union Medical College Press.

Shi Y and Wang G. 2009. *Palliative Medicine Theory and Life Care Practice*. Shanghai: Shanghai Popular Science Press, pp. 29, 35, 57, 72.

Shi Y and Wang G. 2010. *Status and Policy Research of Hospice in Urban China*. Shanghai: Shanghai Science and Technology Education Press, pp. 5–8.

Wang C. 1998. Reflections on the establishment and development of hospice care with Chinese characteristics. *Chinese Medical Ethics* 5: 59–62.

Wang P and Li H. 2005. *Death and Medical Ethics*. Wuhan: Wuhan University Press.

World Health Organization. 2007. *Cancer Control Knowledge into Action: WHO Guide for Effective Programs*. Switzerland: World Health Organization.

World Health Organization. WHO definition of palliative care. Available at: http://www.who.int/cancer/palliative/definition/en/

CHAPTER NINE

MEDICAL FUTILITY IN KOREA

Ivo Kwon

SUMMARY

With the aging of the society and the increasing availability of modern medical practice, end-of-life issues and decisions about medical futility are becoming a critical problem in Korea. In spite of the big social and cultural changes in Korean society since the twentieth century, the traditional culture still has a strong influence on the current practice regarding end-of-life care. Major end-of-life decisions are still frequently made by the guardian of a patient with the attending physician; however, the concepts of patient autonomy and advance directives are being introduced in Korea. Withdrawal of life-sustaining treatment from patients in irreversible conditions based on their own wishes has been legally permitted since the decision by the Supreme Court in 2010. However, active euthanasia or physician-assisted suicide requested by patients is not permitted for the time being.

INTRODUCTION

The Republic of Korea (Korea) has successfully achieved rapid economic growth as well as political democratization in spite of the sufferings from the colonial period (1910–1945) and the ruins of the Korean War (1950–1953). The healthcare system of Korea has also developed amazingly with its economic growth and technological advancement. Accordingly the life expectancy and other indices of health of ordinary Koreans are so much improved in comparison with those of the past. However, as in other parts of the world, Korea is confronting complicated ethical issues regarding healthcare in highly advanced clinical settings. The most urgent one is surely the difficult decision regarding end-of-life care of patients in irreversible conditions. In the United States and some Western countries, respect for the autonomy of the patient plays an important role in this issue, which is based on their own philosophical perspectives. However, in Korea, the genuine wish of the patient regarding the end-of-life decision may sometimes be overridden by the wish or expectation of the family members who are taking care of the patient (Kim *et al.* 2009). The decision is sometimes complicated because of the economic or other kinds of burden of the family due to the insufficient healthcare benefits provided by the national health insurance system. The traditional concepts of life and death from Eastern philosophies and traditional culture overemphasizing filial piety also play a key role in this matter. Therefore it is never easy to answer the question of how to tackle the end-of-life issues in Korean society. However, it is becoming more and more important to the healthcare providers as well as patients themselves with the rapid increase in the aged population and the expansion of intensive care units and the cases of hospital death. In this article, a brief description of the current healthcare system of Korea and its implications for end-of-life issues are discussed. In addition, traditional philosophies such as Confucianism, Taoism, and Buddhism and their influences on current debates regarding the issues are also explained. Finally, the current legal and institutional framework in Korea for dealing with the end of life in general and medical futility in particular is introduced. The aim of the article is to provide a short but intensive description of the current situation regarding end-of-life issues, including medical futility in Korea.

GENERAL OVERVIEW OF THE KOREAN HEALTHCARE SYSTEM

The life expectancy of Korean people who were born in 2009 is 77.0 years for males and 83.8 years for females. The primary cause of death for Koreans is cancer, which accounted for 28% of the total number of deaths in 2008. The next most common causes are cerebro-vascular accident (11.3%), cardiac disease (8.7%), suicide (5.2%), diabetes (4.2%), chronic bronchial disease (3.0%), traffic accident (3.0%), liver disease (2.9%), pneumonia (2.2%), and hypertension (1.9%). The number of deaths due to cancer rapidly increased (108.6 to 139.5 per 100,000 population) during the last 10 years due to the increase in life span of Koreans. In 2010, 246,700 people died, and the major cause of death of 220,000 was chronic diseases including cancers. The cancers frequently found among Koreans are stomach cancer, liver cancer, colon cancer, breast cancer, and cervical cancer (Ministry of Health and Welfare 2011). According to a survey, 55% of Korean people hope to die at home. However, in 2007, just 60% died at hospital, while 26% died in their own home. More than two thirds of Koreans think that they should do their own decision-making regarding their end-of-life care in the absence of socio-economical burdens on the family. This decreases to 44.9% if such a burden exists (Yun 2009).

In 2011 there were 313 general hospitals, 1,262 secondary hospitals, 27,027 private clinics, and 777 nursing homes in Korea. The number of licensed doctors was about 95,000 in 2007. Korea has adopted a dual healthcare system and practitioners of traditional medicine have national licenses; their number was about 20,000 in 2010. The number of licensed nurses was about 230,000 in 2008 (Ministry of Health and Welfare 2011). The number of institutes specializing in hospice and palliative medicine was 43; however, the rate of use of the institutes among terminal cancer patients was only 9% according to the report of the Bioethics Policy Research Center (BPRC 2010). The government revised the Cancer Management Act in 2010, which loosened the qualification for palliative medicine centers to include traditional medicine practitioners and their institutes. But most designated institutes for palliative medicine are tertiary hospitals which run specialized cancer wards or cancer centers and specialized hospice centers. A number of hospice centers were also established for religious and missionary purposes. The Roman Catholic Church initially began to build up its own hospice centers, and Protestants and Buddhist groups have followed in providing their believers with spiritual services in terminal care.

The gross national income per capita for 2009 was 17,175 USD. The whole national healthcare expenditure was about 60 billion USD in 2007, which took 6.80% of GDP. The rate of public support (by National Health Insurance) of the whole healthcare expenditure which includes the cost of health promotion and other items was 54.9%, and the expense for healthcare per capita was 1,688 USD in 2007. In 2009, 73.5% of the total payment for healthcare was covered by the National Health Insurance Corporation (NHIC) and 26.5% was paid for by the patients themselves (NHIC 2011). The national health insurance system has been employed since 1989 so that all Koreans can benefit from it. The Medical Insurance Act was stipulated as early as 1963, but the implementation was delayed to 1977 due to the lack of a sufficient budget. In 1977 workplace-based medical insurance was introduced to workplaces with more than 500 employees. It was expanded to smaller workplaces in 1981 and 1988. The community-based medical insurance system, which was introduced in 1981 to certain rural regions, was expanded to the whole country in 1989. In 1998, the NHIC was launched by integrating the workplace-based and the community-based medical insurance system.

The NHIC provides health check-up services, cash reimbursement for pregnancy exams, and insurance benefits. The NHIC employs a co-payment system where patients should pay 30–60% of the total medical cost according to the level of healthcare providers that they use (they pay more in secondary or tertiary institutes than in primary clinics) and the region of their residency (they pay more in municipal areas than in rural regions). The average monthly charge per person for the NHIC is about 30 USD. The NHIC collected about 33 billion USD from the insured and spent about 34 billion USD (a negative balance of 1 billion USD) in 2010. But the NHIC covered a part of the total medical cost. The total amount of healthcare expenditure in Korea was 77 billion USD in 2010, and it has been rising rapidly. The gap between the total healthcare cost and NHIC expenditure is filled by various private insurances and the patients' own money. In particular the healthcare cost for old people (over 65 years old) has been rising more rapidly and the portion of the NHIC expenditure on such people is 32% and it has doubled since 2004 (NHIC 2011). In summary, Korea is running a kind of universal health insurance system, but its benefits are insufficient to cover all the necessary healthcare costs. Therefore many Koreans will suffer from the burden of healthcare costs especially in the case of grave diseases. This may distort the decision on end-of-life care in some cases.

ETHICS AND END-OF-LIFE ISSUES IN KOREA

Major Ethical Traditions

Traditionally Korean people highly praise the value of life in "this world" in spite of the many sufferings that they are to experience. The negation of this world is very strange to the Korean mind; the Heaven-Earth dualism or disrespect for the materialistic world is not found in Korean thinking. In a famous Korean legend about the origin of the state, Hwan-Woong, a son of the heavenly god, came to love the Earth and asked his father to go down to the Earth. He married a young woman who had been transformed from a bear through a hard initiation test and fathered a son who became the first king of Korea, Tan-gun. In this story, we note a belief that this world is good enough to attract even heavenly beings, and human life is so precious that even animals want to get it. Although Korean people have experienced many invasions by foreign powers, civil wars, famines, and harsh exploitation by the ruling classes through history, the positive attitude and favor for this world has never left the Korean mind. Even in Buddhism, which principally negates the profane values of this world, Korean people created a new sect which is to serve the security and happiness of the human community. Famous Buddhist master Won-Gwang taught five lessons to a warrior group of young nobility of the Silla dynasty (57 BC to AD 935) 1,500 years ago, one of which was "don't kill for an unjustifiable reason". It was different from the teaching of "never kill" preached by other sects. Korean Buddhism is also proud of its tradition of a "monk army" who fought against foreign invaders with fatal weapons. It does not mean that Korean Buddhism permits violence widely. On the contrary, it requires the use of physical violence to be minimized when possible. Together with the concept of in (仁) of Confucianism, it has made the Korean people extremely cautious in taking the life of a human being. Private violence has been strictly banned and murderers should be executed. Even the execution of vicious criminals was prudently permitted only after the review of the king himself. Even a king could not take the life of his people arbitrarily. Another attitude of Buddhism to death is aloofness. Buddhists see life and death as different aspects of one being, with the belief in metempsychosis and karma. The acts conducted in this world will influence the next life, which is due to the logical chain of relationships of every being. In this teaching, there is no room for any transcendental supreme being who presides over the destiny of beings.

Besides Buddhism, which was introduced into Korea during AD 3–4, the Korean mind has also been influenced by shamanism, Confucianism, and Taoism. Shamanism is a very old spiritual legacy from the prehistoric era, and other spiritual traditions came from China and India during the period of ancient kingdoms. The goal of shamanism is to look after the welfare of the people in this world through the mediation of a special person (shaman) with the spiritual beings in that world. The spiritual beings may be the spirits of ancestors, great people, noble animals, or majestic natural phenomena such as high mountains or big rivers. The mission of a shaman is interpreting the will and the revelation of spiritual beings and praying for them to drive off evil and bad things for the welfare of human fellows. Healing patients is one of the major missions of a shaman and shamans served in public hospitals as caregivers with Buddhist monks in ancient times. Health, wealth (with a long life), public honor, and fecundity are blessings sought by shamanism. There has never been a concern for the afterlife in shamanism.

Taoism has been mixed with shamanism in Korea in its search for a long life and health. The original ideal of Taoism preached by Lao-Tsu negated the splendid but hypocritical lifestyle of highly civilized society, and praised instead a simple and humble life that follows the way of nature. However, Taoism was changed into a sort of religion influenced by various sects believed by folks since the Han Dynasty. Alleged Taoist masters (道士) claimed that they had found the secret of life through the investigation of nature. They often wrote prescriptions for diseases and physical weakness (especially lack of sexual energy). It was their ideal to live a life as long as possible in harmony with the order of nature.

Confucianism refuses to mention any supernatural being or phenomenon. In Korea, neo-Confucianism — a new interpretation of Confucianism by Zhu Xi in the twelfth century — was the constructing principle of the Choson Dynasty (1392–1910). Neo-Confucianists were rationalists who denied the existence of any irrational or supernatural beings. Their thoughts and behaviors were based on a very abstract cosmic principle called *li* (理), which is similar to the *logos* of ancient Stoicism. The human mind is a representation of *li* so that it can understand the cosmic principle. The human body itself is a conglomeration of cosmic energy called *ki* (氣), produced by the union of father and mother, and which is dispersed into the universe after death. Human life is precious since it bears *li* in its being. From *li*, filial piety (孝) is derived, a fundamental principle of the morality of Korean neo-Confucianism. It is morally wrong to commit suicide or to injure one's body since such acts would disrespect the parents and are against the ideal of filial piety. However, those acts were sometimes permitted or even praised when they were done for the purpose of the parents, or "bigger parents", i.e. the family, clan, or the state. Bearing a child is an obligation to fulfill the filial piety to the parents or even ancestors. Neo-Confucianists thought death to be a very natural phenomenon, so a wise man should accept it. Death without suffering after fulfilling all human duties (learning, working, and reproduction) has been thought of as both a celebration and a natural phenomenon. However, the concept of filial piety made it morally admirable to help the parents live as long as possible. In certain cases, therefore, a man who lost his parents was blamed as a "sinner" and had to do penance for his "sin" for some time. On the contrary, people had no moral obligation regarding the life of their children; their lives could be sacrificed for the purpose of the whole family. Infanticide was sometimes practiced when the newborn had some physical defects or "unwanted gender", i.e. a girl.

The concepts and customs of neo-Confucianism still have a strong influence on the daily life of Korean people, especially regarding the issues of life and death. The unique combination of aloofness and preoccupation with one's own life in this world, the strong preoccupation with the health and life of one's own parents (which is actually related to the concern about one's own social evaluation for one's performance of filial piety), and relative indifference to the life of one's own child characterize the attitude of Korean people to the issues of life and death (Han *et al.* 2004). Of course, Korean people are experiencing many social and cultural changes today with the urbanization and modernization of society. The value of individual human rights and one's own autonomy is being more and more recognized.

Traditional Health Customs and Culture

The way of using healthcare services, which is colored with traditional practices and customs, is also critical to the understanding of end-of-life issues in Korea. In traditional medicine, the patient should transfer all necessary decisions regarding his own care to his guardian, usually the first son. He had to focus on only "the recovery", and other issues distracting his attention from this final goal were considered bad. Mentioning his prognosis or saying the word "death" was a serious taboo and should be avoided. The duty of the guardian was to do his best to care for his ill parent. Very often, caring for an ill parent was the best practice of filial piety, showing that the guardian had done everything to accomplish this noble duty. As diagnoses were so ambiguous and qualified doctors were so rare in ancient times, "doctor shopping to find a more authoritative one", "getting a second opinion", and "finding a precious medicine" were common. We find such practices still prevalent today.

Sometimes the guardian is afraid of the parent dying outside the home. It has been thought that "good death" is dying at home surrounded by family and friends without any regret. If death occurred outside the home, the family had to find the remains of the dead and bury them at the familial cemetery where the ancestors were buried. Otherwise, the resentment of the dead was believed to give rise to harm or misfortune to the family. It must be noted that the concept of *feng shui* (風水), a belief that the location of one's house or cemetery in the natural environment will have an influence on one's and one's offspring's fortune in the future, has had a strong impact on the Korean mind since ancient times. Hence a "good death at home" and a "good burial" are regarded as very important in one's life. This reluctance towards death outside the home has been used to justify the request of the family to discharge the terminal patient to his home. Before the intervention of legal jurisdiction, physicians used this to justify their decision when a guardian asked them to discharge the terminal patient home for this reason. The concept of a "good death in Korean style" is also found in other issues of end-of-life care. The traditional concept requires all the children to witness their parent's death and the attending physician should keep the patient's body "alive" even after he is already "dead", to wait for the arrival of all his children. It would be a big regret for Korean people not to attend their parent's death. In this context, neglecting a do-not-attempt-resuscitate order or delaying the time of death is also required when waiting for all family members to gather.

A "good burial" is another important issue. Injury to the body of the dead is considered disrespectful to the dead. The body should be buried in earth without any damage and following the right procedures in order for the dead to participate in the circulation of the universe. Nowadays, the number of cremation cases is increasing due to the shortage of cemetery space, but a burial is still preferred. The concept of *feng shui* reinforces such a custom. Autopsy is very rarely done except for legally compromising cases for it is thought to kill the dead a second time. The number of organ donations from brain-dead donors is very low compared with that from living donors in Korea, the reason for which is the hesitation in injuring the body of the dead. Connecting tubes or lines to dying persons appears insulting and disrespectful for they might damage the integrity of the body. Fear of an extraordinary life after such treatment could be partly due to this view.

MEDICAL FUTILITY: ETHICAL GUIDELINES AND REGULATIONS

Professional Codes of Ethics in Korea

The discussion of end-of-life issues used to be a taboo until the late twentieth century in Korea. Preserving the patient's life in any condition was an ethical duty of the physician and the patient's family. Other arguments had hardly ever been suggested to criticize this imperative. But in the

1990s, with the increase in the elderly population, terminal cancer patients, and life-sustaining treatments in ICUs of hospitals, the issue of end-of-life care decisions became an urgent problem that the medical profession had to confront. The Korean Medical Association (KMA) revised the old code of ethics in 1997 to include the following phrase: "A physician should try to relieve the physical and mental sufferings of the terminal patient and help him accept his death with dignity and in an affirmative way." In this code, the acceptance of death "with dignity and in an affirmative way" was first formulated. This concept was epochal to the spirit of Korean physicians who had been taught that they had to fight against disease and death by doing their best. The code of ethics was paraphrased in the Ethical Guidance for Physicians in 2001. Article 28 of the Guidance mentioned the request for discharge against medical advice by the patient himself or his guardian. The article reflected the consequences of the legal dispute in 1997 where a team of neurosurgeons were accused of aiding murder by permitting the discharge of a critically ill patient from the ICU at the request of his wife. In this famous Boramae Hospital case, the patient finally died and his wife was accused of murder. The wife and the surgeons were found guilty in the final judgment of the Supreme Court in 2004 for the reason that the patient could have recovered if not discharged from the ICU. Disputes between the physician and the guardian of the patient over his discharge (and quitting the treatment) were not rare in Korean hospitals. The main reason was usually the futility of the treatment and suffering of the patient, but sometimes it was the economic or physical/psychological burden on the guardian and the family. Article 28 denoted this point and said:

"A physician should respond prudently and appropriately to the request of withdrawal of the treatment or discharge against the physician's advice by the patient himself or his guardian. It may be permitted for the physician to accept such a request if it is submitted in a written document by the autonomous decision of the patient after enough explanation and persuasion, even when the condition of the patient is critical. It may be also permitted for the physician to accept such a request by the legal guardian when the patient is not competent to make a decision because of unconsciousness or other grave condition. In such a case, the physician should judge prudently if the request is in accord with the interest of the patient himself."

The next article (Article 29) advised the physician to consult the ethics committees at various levels (hospital, professional society, and the KMA) for a difficult case. Article 30 dealt with the withdrawal of treatment from a patient in an irreversible condition. The article permitted the physician to accept the request of treatment withdrawal from a patient in an irreversible condition by his own decision or by a legal guardian. The Ethical Guidance of 2001 was a milestone for the debate on end-of-life issues among medical professionals in Korea.

In 2002 the Korean Academy of Medical Sciences (KAMS) established a "special committee for reviewing ethical guidance for the withdrawal of life-sustaining treatment from a terminal patient", which drafted guidance for the withdrawal of life-sustaining treatment. The Guidance for Care of Terminal Patients can be summarized in seven points: (1) The autonomy of the terminal patient should be respected. (2) The decision of withdrawal of life-sustaining treatment should be based on the quality of life and best interest of the patient. (3) The judgment about the futility of a certain treatment or procedure should be cautiously made, sometimes after the review of the hospital ethics committee or physician colleagues. (4) The wish of a patient about a do-not-attempt-resuscitation order should be respected. (5) Denial of the use of the ICU to the terminal patient is sometimes ethically permitted. (6) The terminal patient can be transferred to another institute or his home at his own wish. (7) The opinion of the hospital ethics committee or other third parties should be sought when conflicts or debates happen regarding the decision making. The guidance of the KAMS showed well the complicated situation surrounding the decision of withdrawal of life-sustaining treatment from terminal patients in the early twenty-first century: most physicians did not recognize the concept of patient autonomy; withdrawal of life-sustaining treatment was often confused with euthanasia, so futile treatments including unnecessary ICU care were frequently applied to terminal patients at the demand of his family; and a do-not-attempt-resuscitation order taken from the patient was sometimes neglected at the wish of the family members. The guidance was a first-hand answer to these confusions in the clinical environment.

The Code of Ethics and the KMA Guidance on Ethics were entirely revised in 2006 to respond to the rapidly changing social and clinical environment. The Guidance of 2006 articulated the provisions about end-of-life issues in detail. Article 16 of the Guidance is about "medical intervention and its withdrawal from a terminally ill patient", where a physician (1) should do his best to relieve the physical and mental suffering of the terminally ill patient, (2) should do his best to allow the terminally ill patient to accept his death with dignity and in an affirmative way, (3) should not provide the terminally ill patient who is suffering from uncontrolled pain any artificial and active intervention to advance the time of death, and (4) should not provide the patient any information or method helpful for committing suicide. Article 17 permits the physician to accept the requirement of discharge or discontinuance of treatment from the patient himself or his guardian even when such acts may result in the death of the patient. Article 18 permits the interruption of medically futile treatments. The last two articles were meaningful in the clinical environment of Korea where physicians were legally obliged to provide the best medical care until the end point of life of patients. Consequently, those two articles clashed with the juridical view of those days and brought about serious ethical and legal debates.

Those regulations were still of interest among physicians and legal experts until the Mother Kim case broke out in 2008. In this case, Mother Kim, a 76-year-old woman, fell into a persistent vegetative state (PVS) from brain hypoxic injury and maintained her life connected to an artificial ventilator. As her state was judged to be irreversible, her family asked the hospital (Severance Hospital) to withdraw the ventilator treatment but the hospital denied the request. Her family filed a suit to a local court, and the local court decided to permit the withdrawal of the ventilator treatment. The hospital appealed to the High Court, and the final judgment of the Supreme Court affirmed the permission. The hospital disconnected the ventilator from Mother Kim, who lived more than six months instead of getting a withdrawal of futile treatments and finally died in 2010. This case became a big issue among the mass media and general population, and was an epoch in the history of debates about withdrawal of life-sustaining treatment and euthanasia in Korea.

In 2009, when the legal dispute regarding Mother Kim was going on, Severance Hospital and Seoul National University Hospital (SNUH) announced their own guideline (advice) for withdrawal of life-sustaining treatment in response to the high interest of Korean society. The guideline of Severance Hospital classified the level of patients who could ask for a withdrawal of life-sustaining treatment. The first level group is the patient whose death is imminent from brain death or multiple organ failure. The practice of autonomy is impossible and unpractical for this group and the decision of the hospital ethics committee and the consent of the family is enough for withdrawal. The second level group is the patient suffering from an irreversible condition and brain injury, relying on ventilator treatment. For this group the wish of the patient is critical for the withdrawal of life-sustaining treatment, and the consent of the family is also necessary along with the judgment of the hospital ethics committee. The third group is the patient in an irreversible PVS who maintains voluntary respiration. A court decision is necessary for the withdrawal of life-sustaining treatment from this group.

The advice of SNUH was similar to that of Severance Hospital as it classified the patients into four groups and recommended different approaches according to the level. The advice suggested four basic principles in the decision of withdrawal of life-sustaining treatment: (1) More than two physicians should be involved in the decision of irreversibility of a patient's condition. (2) The attending physician should explain sufficiently the interests and harms of therapeutic options employed in the course of terminal treatment. (3) The patient could deny life-sustaining treatment by writing an advance directive when he did not want it. (4) The practice of active euthanasia and physician-assisted suicide must not be permitted (BPRC 2010).

As those guidelines were individually prepared by different hospitals, the medical society of Korea felt it necessary to make a unified guideline for this issue. Therefore, the KMA, KAMS, and the Korean Association of Hospitals (KAH) established a unified guideline for withdrawal of life-sustaining treatment in September 2009. The guideline suggested five principles with regard to the withdrawal: (1) Futile medical treatment could be withdrawn by medical judgment and the request of the patient. (2) The patient should be provided enough information about his condition and prognosis and his decision should be respected. (3) The attending physician should discuss the related issues with the patient and his family members and must consult with other physicians or the hospital ethics committee about the medical judgment regarding life-sustaining treatment. (4) The attending physician and medical team should try to provide appropriate care including hospice care to the patient. (5) Intentional inducing of the death of the patient or physician-assisted suicide should be prohibited. The guideline is limited to patients who are in the terminal stage of dying or in an irreversible PVS. It classifies this group into four levels according to competence of decision making and survivability with/ without life-sustaining treatment.

This guideline has not been actively used in clinical settings because most physicians do not fully recognize its utility and rely on customary practice (Heo 2009). There is another reason that most hospitals don't actively run a hospital ethics committee; training of medical personnel and financial/administrative support are required to overcome the problems.

Juridical Decisions and Social Consensus

The Criminal Law of Korea punishes a person who kills another person even by the wish or the consent of the victim or helps the victim commit suicide (Criminal Law, Article 252). In this context, any act shortening a person's life, bringing death before the time of natural death, is regarded as "murder", and should be punished without any other justifying condition. Korean jurisdiction generally maintains a very strict position on the practice of euthanasia, not to say of murder. Therefore the practice of active euthanasia would be punished even when the motivation is the relief of an untreatable pain or suffering of the patient. Meanwhile, unintentional inducing of death during pain control of a patient in an irreversible condition could be exempt from punishment if informed consent for the procedure is taken. However, withdrawal of life-sustaining treatment from a patient in an irreversible condition has been subject to hot debates among lawyers as well as physicians.

The first legal case of the Boramae Hospital case has already been mentioned. The patient in this case was not in an irreversible condition, but rather in the phase of recovery from brain surgery. So the Supreme Court found the wife and the surgeons guilty. In 2004, a local court found a father guilty who withdrew ventilator support from his son (and consequently killed him) who was suffering from irreversible paraplegia. In 2008, another father was found guilty who took his son, who was suffering from Duchenne muscular dystrophy, from the ICU back home and let him die. However, the court suspended the sentence considering his motivation. The actual judgment of the court about withdrawal of life-sustaining treatment from patients in an irreversible condition was made in February 2008 in the Mother Kim case. A local court of Seoul declared that the meaningless prolongation of life in terminal patients could impair human dignity, the value of which is confirmed in the Constitution, and the physician could withdraw life-sustaining treatment from the patient at his own request. The appeal court affirmed the judgment in 2009 and listed up to four conditions for withdrawal of life-sustaining treatment: (1) an irreversible condition in a patient facing imminent death, (2) the serious and reasonable wish of the patient, (3) life-sustaining treatment only contributing to the delay of death, and (4) practiced only by a physician.

The Supreme Court finally judged the withdrawal of life-sustaining treatment from patients in an irreversible condition as legal in May 2010. The reasons are summarized as follows: (1) The enforcement of life-sustaining treatment for a patient in an irreversible terminal stage of dying would impair human dignity, so in this exceptional condition, respect for the wish of the patient would secure human dignity and the right to pursue happiness as declared in the Constitution. Therefore withdrawal of life-sustaining treatment could be permitted by the autonomous practice of the right to decision making on the basis of human dignity and the right to pursue happiness. In this case, the irreversibility of the condition should be prudently evaluated by the second opinion of other physicians. (2) Advance directives could be regarded as the practice of the right to decide even after the competence of the patient to decide has vanished. The validity of advance directives should be confirmed by documentation. (3) When advance directives are absent, the wishes of the patient could be presumed by other objective references, daily communications with family or friends, response to similar conditions of others, religion, and other factors. (4) With regard to the irreversibility of the patient's condition, it is favorable to ask a special committee (e.g. hospital ethics committee) to make the decision (Kwon and Choi 2009). This judgment was a decisive event to permit withdrawal of life-sustaining treatment from a patient in an irreversible condition in Korea. Following the judgment, the Ministry of Health and Welfare established a special committee to discuss the issue in 2009. The committee was called the Social Consensus Group for Institutionalization of Withdrawal of Life-Sustaining Treatment (SCG), and was composed of public officials, representatives of the National Assembly, representatives of major religions (Protestants, Buddhists, and Roman Catholics), civil activists, lawyers, and ethicists. The SCG finally agreed on four core issues, but confirmed disagreement for two core issues regarding withdrawal of life-sustaining treatment. The agreed issues are:

1) the subject of withdrawal of life-sustaining treatment (terminal patient facing imminent death and PVS patient in terminal stage);
2) the scope of procedures that could be withdrawn (extraordinary life-sustaining treatment such as artificial ventilator);
3) valid advance directives (documentation confirmed after two weeks of deliberation period);
4) the organization for decision making (hospital ethics committee at institution level; a National Ethics Committee for end-of-life care should be established for oversight).

However, the members had different opinions about the issue of presumption of the wish of the patient and proxy decision making. Major groups agreed that the issue of presumption and proxy decision making could be justified on the condition of strict hospital ethics committee review while minor groups protested that such practice would be abused by easily giving up human life. For the necessity of legalization of this issue, 9 of 18 members disagreed (Ministry of Health and Welfare 2010).

The conclusion of the SCG is the official guideline backed up by the government authority responsible for the issue of withdrawal of life-sustaining treatment in response to the decision of the Supreme Court.

In this procedure, advance directives and hospital ethics committees will play a key role. Therefore the Bioethics Policy Research Center designated by the Ministry of Health and Welfare of Korea started a public campaign introducing advance directives to hospitals and patients in 2010. With the rapid aging of the Korean society, such a campaign drew public attention among those interested in the issue of comfortable dying ("dying well"). It is expected that advance directives and hospital ethics committee reviews will be transferred to the clinical setting in Korea in time.

DECISION-MAKING PROCESS IN THE CASE OF FUTILE TREATMENT IN KOREA

In Korea, withdrawal of futile treatment from a dying patient is understood as enabling "death with dignity", which means facing one's own death in harmony with the order (way) of nature. Before 1997 when the Boramae Hospital case broke out, it was an ordinary custom for a physician to follow the wishes of the guardian, who was usually the spouse or the first son of the patient in an irreversible condition. If the physician did not provide necessary information regarding the patient's condition frankly, the patient could not help guessing his own condition and his opinion was consequently neglected. The attending physician generally only notified the guardian of the current condition and prognosis. It had been thought cruel for the physician to tell the truth about the prognosis directly to the patient. The duty of the physician was cheering up the patient to give him confidence in his recovery. Because talking about death or the possibility of death had been a taboo, the physician and the guardian of a patient did not mention it in front of the patient. Therefore the physician should discuss the medical decision making with the guardian or family member.

Because the NHIC could not fully cover the whole cost for the care, the patient or guardian had to bear the economic burden relating to the medical care. If the patient was old, usually he did not have a full income and was dependent on his guardian (mostly the first son) for his support and care. In this context, the burden on the family was not small, and the opinion of the family had a priority in medical decision making in the case of futile care. Physicians often struggled with a conflict of conscience when the guardian asked for discharge or withdrawal of life-sustaining treatment from a patient who was not yet in the terminal stage, or by contrast, continuing unnecessary treatments including life-sustaining treatment for a patient in the terminal stage of dying. The commonest reason for the former is the economic burden on the family and difficulty of care giving. In Korea, it is the responsibility or ethical duty of the family to attend to the patient in hospital. Because of the low payment from the NHIC, hospitals cannot afford to hire enough nurses for providing nursing care. The shortage of nursing manpower should be compensated for by the family, mostly women. A daughter or daughter-in-law would usually bear the burden of caring for the patient. If the patient does not have a daughter or daughter-in-law, or if the expected female care giver has no time because of her own job, the family should hire a private nursing aid from their own budget, which is highly expensive even for a middle-class family. Either direct care giving or hiring a nursing aid is very burdensome, especially to the family who has a patient in need of long-term hospitalization. In that case, the family is easily tempted to give up the patient. In the Boramae Hospital case, the wife of the patient, who could hardly manage at home with her own labor and small income, was terrified by the prospect of unlimited care giving to her disabled husband without any social support. The surgeons denied her request to discharge her husband several times due to the possibility of his recovery, but finally could not refuse it any more. In recent times, a number of nursing hospitals have been built to accommodate patients who need continuous and supportive care at a modest cost. Still many people feel their ethical responsibility to care for their old and ill parents.

The other extreme phenomenon in contrast with "easily giving up" is the insistence on life-sustaining treatment or even other extraordinary treatments for patients in the terminal stage of dying. As mentioned before, losing one's parents is not only the biggest regret (among many Korean words describing the death of a parent, there is an expression meaning "the heaven broke down"), but even a source of social blame or shame for Korean people, especially when he is thought not to have tried his very best to save the life of his parent. Doing one's best to care for one's ill parent has been regarded as the noblest practice of filial piety, which is the most important basic principle in Korean morality. In ancient times, kings used to award a big prize to the person who was famous for caring for his ill parent in spite of all the difficulties. Today, a highly devoted son or a daughter is still praised by society in many ways. Therefore, some people who can afford to pay all the necessary medical costs ask the physician to employ all necessary treatments regardless of their cost to save the life of their parent until the last moment. The concept of futile treatment will be lost in facing this demand of ostentatious filial piety, and every possible procedure will be recruited. It is easier for the physician to follow such a request than the request for discharge. But such a practice of providing rare and expensive health resources such as ICU care to this kind of patient impairs the limited national health resources and uses up resources for other patients with hope of recovery. But the traditional concept of filial piety and consequently respect for the elderly prevents the whole society from discussing reasonably this matter.

In both cases — easily giving up and insistence on treatment in hopeless conditions — the decision making is usually in the hands of the guardian or the family. The wish of the patient could be easily neglected. Physicians cannot help playing a passive role as provider of the related information and following the wish of the guardian except in cases where a sort of legal dispute, say, accusation of murder, is expected. Sometimes it is hard to reach an agreement among the family members with regard to the decision for the patient. It could provoke a conflict among the family members as well as between the family and the medical team. Therefore some physicians ask the family to reach a consensus among themselves. The hospital ethics committee rarely plays an active role in making a decision regarding end-of-life care except in a few institutes. The reasons are that (1) most hospitals lack a hospital ethics committee, trained persons, and other resources for this matter, (2) physicians and other medical personnel have a poor understanding of hospital ethics committees and lack the experience for running them, and (3) most importantly, the decision regarding end-of-life care is considered a very private matter among the family (Kwon *et al.* 2010). It is not easy for anyone, even a physician, to intervene in the process of decision making unless legal issues exist. With the announcement of the Social Consensus Group on this matter in 2010, the Ministry of Health and Welfare pushed hospitals to set up and run hospital ethics committees and support the civil campaign for writing advance directives. These movements are expected to bring about some change in the current practice.

The guidelines in Korea recommend that the decision making regarding end-of-life care should involve the patient, the guardian (or family members), the physician and medical personnel, and the hospital ethics committee. The decision should be a dynamic process respecting the patient's wishes and accepting the opinions of the concerned parties, which is to be endorsed by the hospital ethics committee. For this purpose, more experience in running such ethics committees and more trained experts are necessary.

MEDICAL FUTILITY AND EUTHANASIA IN KOREA

Koreans highly value the lives of all living creatures on the Earth. Intentional killing without any justifiable reason has been always considered a serious sin. Helping people commit suicide for any reason is ethically unacceptable and can be punished by law. In Korea, neither the practice of euthanasia as in the Netherlands and Switzerland nor the so-called "death with dignity" practiced in the state of Oregon will be permitted for the time being. The recent judgment of the court clarified that the intentional hastening of the end point of life should never be permitted. This attitude is somewhat different from that in Japan where a local court listed certain conditions for euthanasia in 1960s, or that in China where the legalization of active euthanasia has been recently suggested. The majority of lawyers or ethicists in Korea do not differentiate active euthanasia from passive euthanasia in morally and legally meaningful ways (Koh 2009). Regardless of the means employed, intentional hastening of the end point of life would not be morally permissible. Interestingly, withdrawal of futile treatment is acceptable to Korean people even if such act finally results in the death of the patient (Sun *et al.* 2009). It is differentiated from passive euthanasia because the former always presumes an irreversible condition of the patient in the terminal stage while the latter does not. Therefore withholding life-sustaining treatment from the patient whose condition is not irreversible would be regarded as passive euthanasia and punished by law even though his suffering is severe. Of course there is a way for the patient to refuse the life-sustaining treatment by his own will and the

Constitution confirms the right to refuse it. However, for the patient whose condition is too grave to clarify his own wish it should be admitted that a wide ambiguous area remains.

Withdrawal of life-sustaining treatment from the patient in an irreversible condition is understood as enabling "death with dignity" in Korea, which is different from the usage of the term in the US. "Death with dignity" in Korea is not associated with hastening the time of death; rather it means following the natural order of things, free from a low desire to live. The concept of dignity in this context means to behave in a gracious way as a human or to be courageously aloof to death. It would harm the dignity of a person to sustain life in an unnatural and inhumane way by relying on artificial means such as a ventilator and monitoring system. Following the natural order of things is an essential virtue of a learned, enlightened person; he must be aloof to any fear of death and show a calm and stoic attitude when facing death. "Knowing the time of death" is the sign of a really virtuous person who has controlled himself and prepared for his own death throughout his whole life. Therefore advance directives are often understood among Korean elders as the sign of virtue showing that the person is ready for death without any fear.

It is sometimes difficult to distinguish between hastening death and not delaying death in clinical practice. The former would be condemned as euthanasia while the latter accepted as "death with dignity". For this reason, a prudent judgment is really critical and a hospital ethics committee or other institutions should participate in the judging process.

CONCLUSION

In Korea, with the long life expectancy of the population, availability of modern medical care such as ICUs as well as nursing facilities, and an aging population, the issue of end-of-life care is becoming a critical problem. Although a lot of social and cultural changes are occurring with the rapid modernization of Korean society since the twentieth century, the traditional culture and practice still has a strong effect on the current practice regarding end-of-life care including withdrawal of futile treatment from the patient in an irreversible condition. Major decisions are still frequently made by the guardian of a patient with the attending physician;

however, the concept of patient autonomy and the practice of advance directives are being introduced. Withdrawal of life-sustaining treatment from patients in irreversible conditions based on their own wishes has been legally permitted since the decision by the Supreme Court in 2010.

However, active euthanasia or physician-assisted suicide only for the purpose of the best interest or quality of life of a patient has never been and will not be permitted for the time being. Withdrawal of futile treatment from a dying patient is understood as enabling "death with dignity" in Korea, which means facing one's own death in harmony with the order (way) of nature. In this context, writing advance directives means showing one's own virtue in confronting one's death in a stoic and in a different way or showing concern over the burden on the family in providing care, rather than exercising the patient's own autonomy.

REFERENCES

Bioethics Policy Research Center. 2010. *Report on Current Debates and Outlook of the End of Life Issues.* Seoul: BPRC.

Han SS, Um YR, Ahn SH *et al.* 2004. *Nursing Ethics*, Second Edition. Seoul: Korean Nurses Association.

Heo DS. 2009. Patient autonomy and advance directives in Korea. *Journal of Korean Medical Association* 52: 865–870.

Kim SY, Kang HH, Koh YS, and Koh SO. 2009. Attitudes and practices of critical care physicians in end-of-life decisions in Korean intensive care units. *Korean Journal of Medical Ethics* 12: 15–28.

Koh Y. 2009. Physician's role and obligation in the withdrawal of life-sustaining management. *Journal of Korean Medical Association* 52: 871–879.

Kwon I and Choi JY. 2009. The current debates and social trends regarding euthanasia and the withdrawal of life sustaining treatment in Korea. *Korean Journal of Medical Ethics* 12: 127–142.

Kwon I, Koh YS, Yun YH *et al.* 2010. A study on the attitudes of the patients, their family members and physicians toward the treatment withdrawal from the terminal patients in some general hospitals of Korea. *Korean Journal of Medical Ethics* 13: 1–16.

Ministry of Health and Welfare. 2010. *Final Report of the Social Consensus Group on the Withdrawal of Life Sustaining Treatment.* Available at:

http://www.mw.go.kr/front/al/sal0301vw.jsp?PAR_MENU_ID=04&MENU_
ID=0403&BOARD_ID=140&BOARD_FLAG=00&CONT_
SEQ=238554&page=1.

Ministry of Health and Welfare. 2011. *100 Statistical Indices in Health and Social Welfare*. Available at: http://stat.mw.go.kr/stat/content/content_view.jsp?menu_code=MN02040000.

National Health Insurance Corporation. 2011. *Major Statistics of NHIC*. Available at: http://www.nhic.or.kr/portal/site/main/menuitem.9046c7b1fca1aa404bf15151062310a0.

Sun DS, Chun YJ, Lee JH *et al.* 2009. Recognition of advance directives by advanced cancer patients and medical doctors in a hospice care ward. *The Korean Journal of Hospice and Palliative Care* 12: 20–26.

Yun YH. 2009. Hospice-palliative care and social strategies for improvement of the quality of end of life. *Journal of Korean Medical Association* 52: 880–885.

CHAPTER TEN

MEDICAL FUTILITY FROM THE SWISS PERSPECTIVE

Tanja Krones and Settimio Monteverde

SUMMARY

In the past three decades, the debate about medical futility became highly influential in the international bioethics discourse and also in Switzerland. In our contribution, we comment on the ethical debate from our perspective and link our observations to the Swiss healthcare system. We explain its relevance in two pragmatic situations at the beginning and end of life and compare discussions and practices in the US and Germany with discussions and practices in Switzerland. Until now, in the Swiss context decisions about medical futility have taken place predominantly with regard to treatment decisions for particular patients. We describe and critically comment on the "Swiss approach" to futility entailing societal and economic elements of evaluation jointly with a strong reliance on risk-benefit assessments by individual physicians.

INTRODUCTION

In writing our contribution, we first thought about what we consider a valuable aim of dealing with an important medical ethics issue in a cross-cultural perspective in general. It not only touches on recent debates on empirical bioethics (Gabbay *et al.* 2010; Jecker 2007), but also intercultural and global bioethics, dealing with fundamental meta-ethical questions such as the (never-ending and never-solvable) universalism/particularism debate on the one hand and highly practical clinical and public health issues such as cross-border migration, global justice or culturally influenced illness perceptions on the other. Cross-cultural perspectives can both hint at concepts, values and principles being almost universally shared, and point at "national" and "cultural" differences in order to scrutinize values hidden in concepts assumed to be objective or universal, such as medical futility. We decided to first give a short summary of our own view on the futility debate that first came up in the US in the late 1980s because we think that the international bioethics discourse is still very much influenced by US national debates.

We will then give a short overview of the Swiss healthcare system and describe how the concept of futile treatment is dealt with in our country. To investigate the (possible) specifics of the "Swiss way" (albeit being aware of naïve concepts of cultural causal determinants) we chose two paradigmatic cases/situations at the beginning and end of life, treatment of premature infants and do-not-resuscitate (DNR) orders and compared discussions and practices in the US (with regard to premature infants, also Germany) with the discussions and practices in Switzerland.

We thus try to review international similarities and differences in the use of the concept of medical futility as an argument to withhold or withdraw treatments that are not considered to accomplish established purposes or desired outcomes.

The Interplay Between Facts and Values in the Discussion on Medical Futility

As already stated in our introduction and elsewhere in this book the recent debate on medical futility started in the US in the late 1980s. Bioethics was no longer a marginal scientific discipline but had become more influential not only in the medical field but in the whole societal and political sphere. Ethical committees, institutional review boards and professional

codes ruling ethical conduct were visible signs of an ongoing institutionalization. Bioethics not only fostered ethical reflection in the field of
medicine, but — through its institutions — it also exercised a form of
power and control over decision- and policymakers (Engelhardt 2007,
p. 118; Gehring 2004, p. 99).

One of the more general impacts of the new academic field was the
awareness of patient autonomy — not only promoting autonomy without
any costs but concomitantly limiting physicians' influence on medical decision making. The "new" bioethics replaced the "old Hippocratic" ethic of
"doctor knows best," of physicians acting in the patient's best interest,
based only on professional judgments of harms and benefits for the patient.

As most authors today agree (Marco *et al.* 2000; Bishop *et al.* 2010;
Feen 2010) the debate on medical futility first was a kind of reaction to
the rapid rise of patient autonomy and to the question of how patient
autonomy is related to clinical judgment. Second, the first phenomena of
resource scarcity in healthcare settings became visible. Technical and
pharmaceutical advances led to increased demand which was contrasted
by limited supply. It appeared necessary to discriminate between an
appropriate use and an unjustified (and therefore futile) use of life-sustaining or -prolonging means (Kuczewski 2004; Schneiderman 2011). The
debate can be considered as an attempt to spell out the limits of weighing
and specifying patients' autonomy on the one hand and physician-assessed
benefits and harms on the other in the sense of Beauchamp and Childress's
methodology of dealing with conflicting principles (Beauchamp and
Childress 2009). The question posed was whether there is a limit to what
patients may demand: if there are situations in which the physician, relying on her professional judgment of the situation, can refuse to provide a
treatment and justify her decision on the futility of the treatment itself or
of the circumstances in which the treatment is given.

During the following years, many attempts were made to define medical
futility, its concept, content and scope. Whereas there is wide agreement
on the definition of a treatment being futile if it does not "serve its purpose", more specifically if "it cannot benefit the patient" (e.g. Gatter and
Moskop 1995, p. 191), an agreement on what counts as non-beneficial
treatment has not been achieved. All definitions either refer to defining
medical futility via odds (numbers/prognosis of chances) or ends
(observed or prognosticated ends regardless of odds; states that are not

considered as justifying the efforts), that is quantitative or qualitative aspects, which can also be (and are often, especially in practical medical discussions) combined (Jecker 2007).

Brody and Halevy (1995) reflected upon different futile ends defined as follows:

- physiologic futility, when there is no physiologic response to treatment, e.g. no heart action or sufficient blood pressure after resuscitation;
- imminent demise futility, when death in the very near future is expected, e.g. because of organ failure and no possibility for transplantation or replacement of organ function is given;
- lethal condition futility, when a known illness such as cancer will lead to near death;
- qualitative futility, when no acceptable quality of life results from further treatment, e.g. intolerable pain not sufficiently being able to be treated except by deep palliative sedation.

These four defined ends are ordered from narrower to wider scopes of what may count as a futile treatment, the narrowest one being physiologic futility, with no response or possibility of even physiologic reaction, and the widest one being qualitative futility.

Depending on which ends are endorsed/adopted, life-prolonging treatment including CPR may be judged to no longer represent a realistic or appropriate treatment. The authors did not make any ethical judgments on the acceptability of these concepts, nor did they consider probabilities: no odds are mentioned, all ends are assumed to be certain. Although it is helpful to define the content, to ignore the odds is unrealistic. We almost never have 100% certainty in individual cases, not even with regard to physiologic futility.

One of the most oft-cited definitions of medical futility is that of Schneiderman *et al.* (1990) which refers to both probabilities and goals. In their definition a treatment is futile if

a) empirical data suggest a less than 1% chance of success;
b) it merely preserves permanent unconsciousness;
c) it fails to end total dependence on intensive medical care.

Via their definition they criticized both the attempts to define medical futility as mere physiologic futility and to defend the concept of futility as a value-free definition (thus asserting that there is no danger of subjective bias). For them, to define futility as physiologic futility of organ function and not as a sensible outcome for patients is also a value judgment.

This definition, although widely used, has also been criticized. One critique deals with the fact that Schneiderman *et al.* referred to odds and ends but did not combine them directly as odds of permanent unconsciousness or of total dependence on intensive medical care. As already Caplan (1996) has noted, all useful futility judgments contain odds and ends. Regarding the scope of futility, for those who claim physiologic futility to be the only defensible concept to widely include demands for treatment by patients and relatives into the decision-making process (e.g. Truog 2010) the definition is far too wide (and thus might promote undue paternalism). For others, this definition seems much too narrow, since it only focuses on intensive care situations and not, for instance, on situations of terminally demented or incapacitated patients in nursing homes in which some treatments such as invasive procedures and operations may be considered futile (Mols *et al.* 2011).

However, behind these discussions there is another more or less hidden agenda at the root of the futility debate: the consideration of cost effectiveness and just allocation of resources in individual cases. In Beauchamp and Childress's (2009) principlist approach to medical ethics, these dimensions represent the fourth principle of justice, besides autonomy, beneficence and non-maleficence. Justice in the distribution of healthcare resources has almost been neglected in the medical-ethical debates of the 1970s and 1980s. But during the past 20 years major changes occurred: health economics and comparative effectiveness research called for epidemiologic study evidence of aggregated utilities of groups of patients to be considered the most valuable scientific basis for decision making. These approaches have become influential on the individual and political level. They are intensively discussed now at the international level (Gutzwiller *et al.* 2012, p. 10).

Treatment of individual cases is no longer a sphere free of societal implications. Nowadays, the fair allocation of scarce resources, the problem of opportunity costs and the pros and cons of implicit bedside rationing are publicly debated. The tension between individual physicians who allocate resources on the micro level of particular patients and rationing measures introduced on the macro level of policymakers, insurers and providers is overt. It fuels the recent debate on futility. Today, the question of futile treatment is no longer only a question of individual prognosis, risks and benefits in the "intimate" context of the patient-doctor encounter. Nor is it only an expression of professional bodies to prevent the misuse of medicine for unrealizable hopes and desires and to restore physicians' integrity. More and more, the question of futile treatment is linked to the question of wasting limited healthcare resources.

Table 1 summarizes the main pro and con arguments of a wider physician-defined concept of futility that are present in the discussion.

As Gatter and Moskop (1995, p. 193) state: "most commentators agree that proposed definitions of medical futility are appeals to societal consensus on questions of value." The insight that even the decision of only relying on the concept of physiologic futility is already a value decision underlines the necessity to make national differences in concepts of futile treatment explicit. This may contribute to a more thoughtful, transparent approach of defining treatments as "not serving their purpose." Given the value character of these claims about medical futility, we contend that these kinds of judgments have an intrinsically moral nature. They are part of a moral argument, which conclusion (a given treatment should not be carried out) is valid when supported by factual and moral premises that are reasonable.

Table 1.   Pro and Con Arguments of Physician-Defined Wider Concepts of Futility.

Pro arguments	Contra arguments
Physicians must be able to make unilateral value judgments on grounds of their professional integrity and expertise to serve patients best	Unilateral value judgments of physicians in controversial cases may encourage medical paternalism and lead to refusal of treatment for certain groups of people, unduly restricting autonomy and care
Physicians are responsible for stewardship of scarce resources and futile treatment is a waste of resources which impedes efforts to save other patient lives	Empirical studies show different results regarding success rates of various treatments; an absolute clear definition of futile treatment is not easy
Empirical evidence suggests that some treatments have very low success rates	No societal consensus exists (also not among physicians) about appropriate success rates or valuable treatment goals

SALIENT FEATURES OF THE SWISS HEALTHCARE SYSTEM

For about 20 years, the Swiss healthcare system has been subject to important transitions in response to epidemiological and demographical challenges also faced by other medically highly developed countries (OECD/WHO 2011). Since the enactment of the Health Insurance Law in 1996, all residents are obliged to contract and obtain basic insurance coverage with a health insurance company. The insurance is not related to occupational status. Therefore, also the unemployed have to pay for it (Reinhardt 2004).

Together with the tradition of cantonal and municipal autonomies, the political structure of direct democracy implies a high participation of the electorate also for healthcare matters. Not only the federal acts concerning transplantation medicine, abortion, human research, reproductive medicine and public health are submitted to public scrutiny. There are also comparatively low thresholds to influence ongoing and completed legislation through a large right of referendum and initiative. Departing from a basically free market and choice-based system with extensive executive powers at the cantonal level, these changes consist mainly in reshaping healthcare policies by redefining, redistributing or transferring regulative, distributive and executive powers between the main protagonists of the Swiss healthcare system (Kocher 2010): the Confederation, the 26 sovereign cantons, the municipalities, insurers, consumers, providers, the healthcare workforce, the pharmaceutical and medical technical industry.

The aim of these changes to the structure of the Swiss healthcare system was to meet different healthcare needs for individuals, the population and society in times of relative healthcare resource scarcity. Within this framework of fast-changing social conditions for the provision of healthcare, reflections on medical futility are seldom explicitly addressed. Nevertheless, such reflections can be detected in different domains which are horizontally and vertically interconnected:

- the level of public healthcare policy and legislation (Health Insurance Act of 1996 and respective by-laws and amendments, cantonal healthcare law);

- the level of profession-specific evidence-based practice guidelines (professional bodies such as the Swiss Medical Board);
- the level of professional ethics (guidelines of the Swiss Academy of Medical Sciences).

Consensus and Controversies

Departing from different standpoints, consensus emerges that — in the Swiss context of a high-tech, high-quality, high-cost and personnel-intensive healthcare supply — it is a political, legal and moral imperative to avoid or reduce any medical treatment under futile conditions (Daley and Gubb 2007; Oggier 2010). Beyond this consensus there is a fundamental disagreement about how the different stakeholders can best achieve this objective. The following proposals have been discussed nationwide by professional bodies, political parties and authorities:

- fostering preventive medicine (see OECD/WHO 2011);
- optimizing the interface between federal and cantonal law (Achtermann and Berset 2006);
- fostering models of managed care by limiting choice of provider (see Baumberger 2010; after the successful making of the legal initiative, the statutory introduction of managed care will be submitted to a popular vote in September 2012);
- fostering a better stratification of risks by enforcing a single statutory insurance (first rejected by the Swiss electorate in 2007, new legal initiatives are pending).

Although these approaches do not mutually exclude each other, each of them has implications for the traditional Swiss healthcare landscape in the process of reshaping roles, rights and duties of the aforementioned protagonists.

MEDICAL FUTILITY AT THE BEGINNING AND END-OF-LIFE IN SWITZERLAND COMPARED WITH THE UNITED STATES

How decisions are made and treatment limits set with regard to preterm babies with extremely low birth weight is not only influenced by concepts of medical futility (or utility). It is also linked to more general dimensions such as dignity, limits of "utilitarian arguments" regarding the "value of life," the status of embryos and fetuses, and the rights of women and parents to decide for their children and family life — before and after birth. Yet, how and when limits are set with regard to life-prolonging treatment of babies born at very low gestational age and weight also serves as an illustrative example of the underlying concept of medical futility. The question of "how small is too small" was always linked to all concepts of futility — from physiologic futility to quality of life futility. As the development of treatment of very low birth and gestational age infants shows, the presumably "objective, physiological" border of futility — defined as the viability of very preterm children — has moved. Whereas in the 1960s and 1970s, viability was set at about seven months such as in the famous Roe *et al.* v. Wade decision of the US Supreme Court on abortion (US Supreme Court 1973), and a birth weight under 1,000 g was considered critical for viability, the limit is now much lower with regard to gestational age and weight. "Miracle babies," most of them born in the US but also Germany and other countries (Japan, Romania), survived at a gestational age of 21+ weeks and less than 300 g. It is also a well-known fact that rates of survival of preterm infants differ internationally and across European countries (Zeitlin *et al.* 2008) and that decisions to forgo life-sustaining treatment is most often made before patients die, in the neonatal intensive care unit (NICU) as well as in intensive care units of adult patients. Thus, although other factors (skills, transportation, prevention and treatment in pregnancy) might contribute to these "hard facts," different values are clearly an important influence factor in what counts as a futile treatment, resulting for instance in decisions not to resuscitate a child immediately after birth and when to involve parents into the decision-making process.

The differences are visible both in guidelines and practice. It is not by chance that some of the youngest and smallest children were born in the US and Germany. In these countries, guidelines suggest life-prolonging treatment at a gestational age of 23 weeks or even less (Table 2).

As Table 2 demonstrates, there are not only remarkable differences with regard to thresholds but also with regard to the inclusion of parents' values and wishes into the decision-making process.

In all three countries, guidelines were recently revised, interestingly placing less absolute limits regarding thresholds except for the upper limit of parent involvement in the German guideline, where the best interest of the child ("non-futility"to"utility" to "best interest of the child") is assumed to prevail at 24 0/7 weeks of gestational age.

In Switzerland, the limit of life-prolonging care was set at 23 6/7 weeks until last year (Berger *et al.* 2002; Berger *et al.* 2011). Parents' involvement remains an important issue but previously was only accepted as a decisional factor from the 24th gestational week (24 0/7) besides the risk-benefit evaluation of physicians. Below the gestational age of 23 6/7 weeks only comfort care was considered appropriate, and parents had no official say with regard to life-prolonging treatment up to this gestational age.

The new Swiss guidelines entail general first- and second-order risk-benefit evaluations by physicians. No life-prolonging treatment is offered

Table 2. Guidelines for Forgoing Life-Sustaining Treatment and Involving Family Members in the Decision.

Parameter	US[1]	Germany[2]	Switzerland[3]
Absolute threshold of no life-sustaining treatment (physicians' decision only)	Not given any more Reference to the Nuffield Council on Bioethics (22 0/7 weeks)	22 0/7 weeks Not absolute, "as a rule no resuscitation"	23 0/7 to 23 6/7 weeks Palliative care as a rule, parents' wishes included if positive prognostic factors prevail
Involvement of parents regarding life-sustaining treatment	From the very beginning	22 0/7 to 23 6/7 weeks Involvement of parents' views	24 0/7 to 24 6/7 weeks Parents' wishes included and evaluated
Absolute threshold of life-sustaining treatment (physicians' decision only)	Not given any more Reference to the Nuffield Council on Bioethics (24 0/7 weeks), parents still involved	24 0/7 weeks Best interest of the child	25 0/7 to 25 6/7 weeks Parents' wishes included if negative prognostic factors are prevalent

1. Batton *et al.* (2009); 2. AWMF (2007); 3. Berger *et al.* (2011).

to children below 23 0/7 weeks, which means a shift of several days in the absolute limit (from 23 6/7 to 23 0/7 weeks) compared to the previous guidelines. Above 23 0/7 weeks parents are allowed and encouraged to be part of the decision-making process, but this depends on the first- and second-order evaluation of physicians. In general, comfort care is proposed until the gestational age of 23 6/7 weeks. Only if there are additional ("objective") positive prognostic factors, parents are invited to decide whether, contrary to the general approach of offering comfort care, life-prolonging care is appropriate. Parents are further invited to participate in all decisions for their children if they are born between 24 0/7 and 24 6/7 gestational weeks. In all of these children, intensive care is cautiously offered ("provisional intensive care"), positive and negative prognostic factors are evaluated and decisions made by physicians and parents in a shared decision-making process. From 25 0/7 weeks onwards, intensive care is a rule and parents are only invited to decide on forgoing life-prolonging care, if there are ("objective") negative prognostic factors.

Compared to guidelines from Germany and the US, one can conclude that the border of medical futility is quantitatively placed later in Switzerland with regard to viability and futile treatment of very preterm newborns. The concept of futility is also qualitatively "wider" with regard to both odds and ends: a qualitative concept of futility according to the definition of Brody and Halevy (1995) with far wider odds than the definition of Schneiderman *et al.* seems to underlie the Swiss concept of futile treatment of these patients. Remarkably, the decision to forgo life-sustaining treatment of very preterm newborns is clearly defined as a value decision, in which societal, economical and legal elements are also important criteria.

Excursus: Guidelines as Culturally Embedded Constructs

Societal or economic factors influencing the process of guideline preparation are not mentioned in the US and German guidelines. This might be attributed to the fact that the evaluation of economic factors has always been an important element of Swiss healthcare policy due to decentralized patterns of responsibility that reflect the interests of different stakeholders (Federal Office of Public Health 2005):

- the 26 sovereign cantons and their fundamental role in healthcare legislation, execution, governance of supply and demand and monitoring of costs (the insurance rates for the same coverage being different from one canton to another);
- the subsidiarity of federal law;
- high deductibles of statutory health insurances for patients and incentives for elective cost containing insurance models (managed care models like health maintenance organizations);
- the historically transmitted Swiss policy tradition, that holds the citizens' opinion to be of importance for every aspect of societal life and therefore to be considered and incorporated in the process of establishing policies.

Compared to the US guideline, the Swiss guideline relies on wider ("objective") utility assessments by the physician. First, it clearly places more decisional power on professional judgments regarding the decision to forgo life-sustaining treatment against parents' wishes for children with "better" probabilities and likely outcomes. Second, it gives no more limits and centrally involves parents in every decision. It thus defines even narrow physiologic futility ("absolute viability") as a value-laden decision where parents are to be involved. The German guideline also only partly involves parents in the decision-making process compared to the US guideline, yet the decision-making power of parents is limited in a different way: the limit is placed on wishes of parents to forgo life-sustaining treatment, asserting the general "utility" of life-prolonging treatment at 24 0/7 weeks of gestational age, a time at which the US and Swiss guidelines centrally involve parents in an open decision-making process.

For us these "national" and "cultural" differences in defining the viability and futility of treatment of very preterm newborns are not random. They prove our contention that futility has to be seen as a culturally mediated construct that reflects the values that are shared in a particular context. One of the authors (TK) has worked in both Germany and Switzerland and observed practices in NICUs in each of these countries. In the author's personal experience as a clinical ethicist practicing in both Germany and Switzerland, the practices in NICUs are in fact different with regard to these borderline cases. In these cases, German physicians tend to be more optimistic than those in Switzerland. Consequently, parents were encouraged to embrace life-prolonging treatment in Germany, whereas they were more likely to be discouraged from such treatment in similar cases in Switzerland. The observation that in Switzerland, wider, qualitative concepts of medical futility (still) relying on the physicians' judgments of risk and benefit exist, is also partly visible in decisions on end-of-life issues, specifically do-not-resuscitate orders.

Do-Not-Resuscitate Orders in Switzerland

One of the paradigmatic treatments for which medical futility is discussed is cardiopulmonary resuscitation, which also underlies the widely used definitions of medical futility by Brody and Halevy (1995) and Schneiderman *et al.* (1990), see also Ardagh (2000) and Tomlinson *et al.* (1990).

First, compared to the US, do-not-resuscitate orders are less routinely discussed with patients on the one hand, but resuscitation is also routinely performed in patients with a very low chance of success on the other (for data and further references see SAMS 2008, Chapter 1.2.1). In Switzerland, the Swiss Academy of Medical Sciences (SAMS) is in charge of defining most of the medico-ethical and clinical ethical guidelines, many of them supported also by other professional bodies such as the Swiss Nurses' Association. This body of "soft" professional law binds physicians in our country and can be incorporated into "hard" law through fixed or dynamic references (cantonal healthcare laws, federal act on organ transplantation concerning the determination of death). With regard to end-of-life decisions, several important guidelines were published during the last 10 years:

- care of patients at the end of life (SAMS 2004a);
- palliative care (SAMS 2006);
- treatment and care of elderly persons who are in need of care (SAMS 2004b);
- treatment and care of patients with chronic severe brain damage (SAMS 2003);
- decisions on cardiopulmonary resuscitation (SAMS 2008);
- determination of death in the context of organ transplantation (updated guideline, SAMS 2011).

All of these guidelines clearly consider transparency of decisions and autonomy of patients as the most important ethical aspects and principles to consider with regard to end-of-life decisions. In severe brain injuries, the question whether life-prolonging or palliative care is considered appropriate is closely linked to the formerly expressed will of the patient. No defined "physiologic" limit is given with regard to life-prolonging treatment. If there is no clear advance statement of the patient's will or if there is any doubt about it, giving enteral or parenteral food and fluid is considered as being indicated only in patients who have clinically stable vital parameters. Measures should be adapted to therapeutic aims defined together by physicians, patients or their representatives (SAMS 2003). Resuscitation is not mentioned in the guidelines for treating severely brain injured or very old care-dependent patients. In the specific guideline on resuscitation, however, although the wish of the patient with regard to resuscitation is considered one of the most important points for consideration, a limit is given indicating when resuscitation is considered a futile treatment. If death is expected within days or weeks, resuscitation is not considered as being indicated. If the prognosis is not that clear and the life expectancy is considered to comprise several months, the patient's values and preferences are incorporated into the decision-making process clarifying whether resuscitation should be performed or not.

In sum, although the guidelines of the Academy do not exhibit an explicit discourse on medical futility, they implicitly address the topic for different clinical contexts. They affirm the basically value-laden character of such decisions, demand an accurate assessment of the ethical concerns, procedural transparency and the primacy of the patient's will and interests. At the same time, the guidelines establish room for reflection on futility by physicians and other healthcare professionals in charge.

Besides these guidelines, several publications discuss a wider conception of futile treatment. In an article by a Swiss interdisciplinary research group in clinical ethics (Mols *et al.* 2011), the concept of medical futility is thoroughly discussed with regard to wider concepts. Referring to a case of operating on a demented, care-dependent patient, futility is defined as overtreatment also in cases beyond intensive care units contrary to Schneiderman *et al.*'s definition, but leaves open the question about a due "baseline" treatment. Departing from these situations over- and undertreatment can be described. Compared to the debate in the US, again there seems to be a tendency to adopt wider discretional boundaries within the

Swiss healthcare system, in setting limits on treatments identified as "not being indicated". Although highly criticized, the American Heart Association (see Marco *et al.* 2000) defends a concept of physiologic futility with regard to resuscitation. It is considered futile if

a) no survivors have been reported in well-designed studies in given circumstances;
b) basic and advanced life support have been provided without success;
c) no physiological benefit can be expected through performing resuscitation.

Not all American physician associations are that restrictive with regard to setting limits for indicated treatments; some define medical futility as a treatment being "highly unlikely" to result in meaningful survival such as the American College of Chest Physicians (1990). But recent debates such as the one initiated by Truog (2010) on performing resuscitation in children even in clearly futile situations, if parents request CPR, for the purpose of comforting parents and if resuscitative interventions are not harmful, suggest that cultural differences seem to exist also with regard to rationales for performing CPR (Truog *et al.* 1992; Paris *et al.* 2010).

Again, in Switzerland, as compared to the US, when the patient's preferences or interests cannot be clearly established, physicians tend to take the task of setting limits on life-sustaining treatment, concomitantly and implicitly limiting patients' or parents' autonomy by establishing what futility *means* in a given situation (for qualitative data in the critical care setting see Albisser *et al.* 2008).

The Case of Non-Heart-Beating Organ Donation

Very recently, non-heart-beating donation (NHBD) of organs, which was first performed in Switzerland 10 years ago, became possible and was re-initiated in two centers (Zurich and Geneva) due to juridical changes that consisted in an alignment of the Swiss transplantation law and the guidelines of the Academy (SAMS 2011). NHBD is defined via the Maastricht categories, the first and the second referring to unsuccessful (attempts) or useless (heart stopping in brain-dead patients) resuscitation, the third category referring to decisions to forgo life-sustaining treatment in severely ill patients, touching a wider concept of medical futility (Beyeler *et al.* 2009). When the decision is made, life-sustaining treatments (for example ventilator, drugs sustaining circulation such as adrenaline) are withdrawn. If the patient dies within a given time (as a prerequisite that organs can be taken) and death proven by verification of cardiac arrest, organs are retrieved. Often, patients who become eligible for non-heart-beating donation suffer from severe brain injuries. We know that rates, policies and procedures to perform NHBD differ worldwide (Bernat *et al.* 2006; Rady *et al.* 2010). These differences do not constitute a mere technical problem. They reflect fundamental uncertainties about a judgment of medical futility, predominantly in view of the consequences: undoubtedly, continuing life support in these patients would be medically futile. But immediately after declaring them dead by traditional cardiopulmonary criteria, vital organ extraction is performed.

For these reasons, whereas many countries have introduced NHBD programs, some countries such as Germany do not allow NHBD. They fear a slippery slope may develop by withdrawing a life-sustaining therapy considered futile, and declare death in compliance with the dead donor rule and retrieve organs. Although the guidelines of the SAMS impose a "hopeless prognosis" as a necessary condition for patients under this protocol and no capability for survival without a high support of vital functions (SAMS 2011, p. 14), this again sets up a discretional space, hinting at culturally or nationally influenced definitions of medical futility. More research on which situations are considered "futile enough" to forgo treatment and perform NHBD in Maastricht category III might further illuminate the different values behind presumable objective definitions of medically futile treatment.

THE "SWISS APPROACH" TO THE FUTILITY DEBATE

Value judgments are indispensable to scientific practices such as defining research questions, making assumptions, setting significant thresholds, or balancing between the advantages and disadvantages of different methodologies. Scientific knowledge cannot be value free, but this does not make it any less scientific (Petrova *et al.* 2006, p. 705).

The "Swiss approach" to medical futility (if there is anything such as a national way) is by no means a uniform one. Economic constraints make it necessary to contain healthcare expenditures. The measures taken to reach cost containment are situated in a web of the political, the professional, the insurer, and the autonomy of the insured as well as provider. All these measures constitute the framework, in which empirical evidence and values are dealt with and moral arguments underlying statements about medical futility are constructed. Once a treatment is considered medically futile under certain conditions, there is no moral obligation to offer it — even at the patient's request or for other than medically accepted reasons. This is what we mean by the moral nature of futility judgments.

In Switzerland, there is a shift towards increased federal regulation, first inaugurated in 1994 through the enactment of the Health Insurance Law. Article 32 gives a statutory basis to the principles of cost-effectiveness, efficacy and usefulness (Swiss Confederation 2012). With this taxonomy, a conceptual foundation for a nationwide discourse about medical futility has been laid, even though from the narrow viewpoint of the coverage of costs.

In contrast to the origins of the futility debate mentioned earlier in the US, the role of patient autonomy in shaping allocation policies in the case of presumed futility remains unclear. Since the enactment of the Health Insurance Law, different cases about the refusal of insurers or the state to pay interventions deemed medically futile have drawn public attention. In one case that has recently come up before the Federal Supreme Court — the Myozyme™ case — concerning the so-called off-label use of an "orphan drug", the Court ruled that the insurer was not obliged to cover the yearly costs of about 500,000 Swiss francs (545,000 USD). The reasons were, first, that the treatment does not have a substantial therapeutic benefit, and second, the question of cost-effectiveness (for a detailed description see Kesselring 2011).

These days, insurers, providers, patients and the public are involved in an ongoing process of reshaping healthcare policies by promoting patient responsibility through economic incentives, proposing options of managed care and new prospective payment systems for hospitalized patients (Swiss-DRG). Within these transitions, not only the reliability and validity of the concept of medical futility plays a crucial role, but also the way of communicating futility judgments to those individuals who are directly affected by these decisions.

CONCLUSION

Until now, in the Swiss context decisions about medical futility have taken place predominantly with regard to treatment decisions for particular patients. A qualitative, wide concept of medical futility prevails, entailing societal and economic elements of evaluation jointly with a strong reliance on risk-benefit assessments by individual physicians. As mentioned earlier, for compelling reasons of justice and ethical sustainability they have to be justified also at a meso and macro level, shaping the range of therapeutic decision-making discretion with accepted moral standards of the healthcare professionals as expressed in the guidelines of the Swiss Academy of Medical Sciences and/or the Swiss Nurses' Association. It is the substantially moral nature of medical futility judgments which imposes accountability on the criteria adopted and the decisions taken. The characteristic "Swiss way" of reaching this goal — through democratic participation and legitimation — may not be the easiest way but is surely the most preferable when accompanied by measures of public information and education.

REFERENCES

Achtermann W and Berset C. 2006. *Gesundheitspolitiken in der Schweiz — Potential für eine nationale Gesundheitspolitik, Volume 1, Analyse und Perspektiven.* Bern: Federal Office of Public Health.

Albisser Schleger H, Pargger H, and Reiter-Theil S. 2008. Futility, Übertherapie am Lebensende? Gründe für ausbleibende Therapiebegrenzung in Geriatrie und Intensivmedizin. *Zeitschrift für Palliativmedizin* 9: 67–75.

American College of Chest Physicians/Society for Critical Care Medicine Consensus Panel. 1990. Ethical and moral guidelines for the initiation, continuation, and withdrawal of intensive care. *Chest* 97: 949–958.

Arbeitsgemeinschaft der Wissenschaftlichen Medizinischen Fachgesellschaften (AWMF). 2007. Frühgeburt an der Grenze der Lebensfähigkeit des Kindes.

S2 Leitlinie. AWMF Register 024/019 (Preterm birth at the limit of viability of the child Consensus guideline of the German Society of gynecologists, pediatricians, neonatal intensive care and pediatric intensive care). Available at: http://www.awmf.org/uploads/tx_szleitlinien/024–019l_S2k_Fruehgeburt_ Grenze_der_Lebensfaehigkeit-2007–12.pdf [Accessed February 10, 2012].

Ardagh M. 2000. Futility has no utility in resuscitation medicine. *Journal of Medical Ethics* 26: 396–399.

Batton DG for the AAP Committee on Fetus and Newborn. 2009. Clinical report: Antenatal counseling regarding resuscitation at an extremely low gestational age. *American Academy of Pediatrics* 124: 422–427.

Baumberger J. 2010. Managed care. In: G Kocher and W Oggier, eds. *Gesundheitswesen in der Schweiz 2010–2012. Eine aktuelle Übersicht*, Fourth Edition. Bern: Huber, pp. 197–206.

Beauchamp T and Childress J. 2009. *Principles of Biomedical Ethics*, Sixth Edition. Oxford: Oxford University Press.

Berger TM, Büttiker V, Fauchère J-C et al. 2002. Swiss Society of Neonatology guidelines. Recommendation of care for preterm infants at the limit of viability (Gestational age 22–26SSW). Available at: http://www.neonet.ch/assets/doc/ gestationsalter-d.pdf [Accessed February 10, 2012].

Berger TM, Bernet V, El Alama S et al. 2011. Perinatal care at the limit of viability between 22 and 26 completed weeks of gestation in Switzerland. 2011 revision of the Swiss recommendations. *Swiss Medical Weekly* 141: w13280. Available at: http:// www.neonet.ch/assets/pdf/Publication_Limit_of_ Viability.pdf [Accessed February 10, 2012].

Bernat JL, D'Alessandro AM, Port FK et al. 2006. Report of a national conference on donation after cardiac death. *American Journal of Transplantation* 6: 281–291.

Beyeler F, Wälchli-Bhend S, Marti H-P, and Immer F. 2009. Wiedereinführung des Non-Heart-Beating-Donor-Programms in der Schweiz? *Schweizerische Ärztezeitung* 90: 899–901.

Bishop JP, Brothers KB, Perry JE, and Ahmad A. 2010. Reviving the conversation around CPR/DNR. *American Journal of Bioethics* 10: 61–67.

Brody BA and Halevy A. 1995. Is futility a futile concept? *Journal of Medicine and Philosophy* 20: 123–144.

Caplan AL. 1996. Odds and ends: Trust and the debate over medical futility. *Annals of Internal Medicine* 125: 688–689.

Daley C and Gubb J. 2007. *Healthcare Systems: Switzerland.* London: Civitas Institute for the Study of Civil Society. Available at: http://www.civitas.org. uk/nhs/switzerland.pdf [Accessed December 23, 2011].

Engelhardt HT Jr. 2007. Bioethics as politics. A critical reassessment. In: LA Eckenwiler and FG Cohn, eds. *The Ethics of Bioethics. Mapping the Moral Landscape.* Baltimore, MD: Johns Hopkins University Press, pp. 118–133.

Federal Office of Public Health. 2005. *The Swiss Health System,* Second Edition. Bern: Federal Office of Public Health. Available at: http://www.bag.admin.ch [Accessed December 23, 2011].

Feen E. 2010. Leave current system of universal CPR and patient request for CPR orders in place. *American Journal of Bioethics* 10: 80–81.

Gabbay E, Calvo-Broce J, Meyer KB, Trikalinos TA, Cohen J, and Kent DM. 2010. The empirical basis for determinations of medical futility. *Journal of General Internal Medicine* 25: 1083–1089.

Gatter RA and Moskop JC. 1995. From futility to triage. *Journal of Medicine and Philosophy* 20: 191–205.

Gehring P. 2004. *Foucault — Die Philosophie im Archiv.* Frankfurt am Main: Campus.

Gutzwiller F, Biller-Andorno N, Harnacke C *et al.* 2012. *Methoden zur Bestimmung von Nutzen bzw. Wert medizinischer Leistungen* (Methods of assessing the benefits and value of medical interventions). Basel: Swiss Academies of Arts and Sciences.

Jecker NS. 2007. Medical futility: A paradigm analysis. *HEC Forum* 19: 3–32.

Kesselring F. 2011. First fundamental decision of the Federal Supreme Court of Switzerland on cost-effectiveness in the area of human healthcare. *European Journal of Risk Regulation* 3: 442–446.

Kocher G. 2010. Kompetenz- und Aufgabenteilung Bund — Kantone — Gemeinden. In: G Kocher and W Oggier, eds. *Gesundheitswesen in der Schweiz 2010–2012. Eine aktuelle Übersicht,* Fourth Edition. Bern: Huber, pp. 133–144.

Kuczewski MG. 2004. Ethics committees and case consultation. Theory and practice. In: G Khushf, ed. *Handbook of Bioethics. Taking Stock of the Field from a Philosophical Perspective.* Dordrecht: Kluwer, pp. 315–334.

Marco CA, Larkin GL, Moskop JC, and Derse AR. 2000. Determination of futility in emergency medicine. *Annals of Emergency Medicine* 35: 604–612.

Mols AM, Reiter-Theil S, Oertli D, and Viehl CT. 2011. Futility: ein Begriff im chirurgischen Alltag (Futility: A concept of surgical day to day practice?). *Hessisches Ärzteblatt* 8: 478–481.

OECD/WHO. 2011. OECD *Reviews of Health Systems: Switzerland 2011*. Paris: OECD Publishing. Available at: http://dx.doi.org/10.1787/9789264120914-en [Accessed February 20, 2012].

Oggier W. 2010. Kosten und Finanzierung. In: G Kocher and W Oggier, eds. *Gesundheitswesen in der Schweiz 2010–2012. Eine aktuelle Übersicht*, Fourth Edition. Bern: Huber, pp. 157–166.

Paris JJ, Angelos P, and Schreiber MD. 2010. Does compassion for a family justify providing futile CPR? *Journal of Perinatology* 30: 770–772.

Petrova M, Dale J, and Fulford KW. 2006. Value based practice in primary care. Easing the tensions between individual values, ethical principles and best evidence. *British Journal of General Practice* 56: 703–709.

Rady MY, Verheijde JL, and McGregor JL. 2010. Scientific, legal, and ethical challenges of end-of-life organ procurement in emergency medicine. *Resuscitation* 81: 1069–1078.

Reinhardt UE. 2004. The Swiss health system. Regulated competition without managed care. *JAMA* 292: 1227–1231.

Schneiderman LJ. 2011. Defining medical futility and improving medical care. *Bioethical Inquiry* 8: 123–131.

Schneiderman LJ, Jecker NS, and Jonsen AR. 1990. Medical futility: Its meaning and ethical implications. *Annals of Internal Medicine* 112: 949–954

Swiss Academy of Medical Sciences (SAMS). 2003. Treatment and care of patients with chronic severe brain damage. Medical-ethical guidelines. Available at: http://www.samw.ch/en/Ethics/Guidelines/Currently-valid-guidelines.html [Accessed February 9, 2012].

Swiss Academy of Medical Sciences (SAMS). 2004a. Care of patients at the end of life. Medical-ethical guidelines of the SAMS. Available at: http://www.samw.ch/en/Ethics/Guidelines/Currently-valid-guidelines.html [Accessed February 9, 2012].

Swiss Academy of Medical Sciences (SAMS). 2004b. Treatment and care of elderly persons who are in need of care. Medical-ethical guidelines and recommendations. Available at: http://www.samw.ch/en/Ethics/Guidelines/Currently-valid-guidelines.html [Accessed February 9, 2012].

Swiss Academy of Medical Sciences (SAMS). 2006. Palliative care. Medical-ethical guidelines and recommendations. Available at: http://www.samw.ch/en/Ethics/Guidelines/Currently-valid-guidelines.html [Accessed February 9, 2012].

Swiss Academy of Medical Sciences (SAMS). 2008. Decisions on cardiopulmonary resuscitation. Medical-ethical guidelines and recommendations. Available at: http://www.samw.ch/en/Ethics/Guidelines/Currently-valid-guidelines.html [Accessed February 9, 2012].

Swiss Academy of Medical Sciences (SAMS). 2011. The determination of death in the context of organ transplantation. Medical-ethical guidelines. Available at: http://www.samw.ch/en/Ethics/Guidelines/Currently-valid-guidelines. html [Accessed February 9, 2012].

Swiss Confederation. 2012. Health Insurance Act (Schweizerische Eidgenossenschaft, Bundesgesetz vom 18. März 1994 über die Krankenversicherung (KVG). Stand am 1. Januar 2012). Available at: http://www.admin.ch/ch/d/sr/c832_10.html [Accessed February 9, 2012].

Tomlinson T and Brody H. 1990. Futility and the ethics of resuscitation. *JAMA* 264: 1276–1280.

Truog RD. 2010. Is it always wrong to perform futile CPR? *New England Journal of Medicine* 362: 477–479.

Truog RD, Brett AS, and Frader J. 1992. The problem with futility. *New England Journal of Medicine* 326: 1560–1564.

US Supreme Court. 1973. Roe *et al.* v. *Wade*; District Attorney of Dallas County Appeal from the United States District Court for the Northern District of Texas no. 70–18; 410; US 113.

Zeitlin J, Draper ES, Kollee L *et al.* for the MOSAIC study group. 2008. Differences in rates and short term outcome of live births before 32 weeks of gestation in Europe in 2003: Results from the MOSAIC cohort. *Pediatrics* 121: 936–944.

CHAPTER ELEVEN

MEDICAL FUTILITY IN TURKEY

Berna Arda and Ahmet Acıduman

SUMMARY

As a country located between Asia and Europe, Turkey is both a Balkan
and a Middle Eastern country, and is of both Black Sea and Mediterranean
origin. Its culture is based on both Eastern and Western thought. It is an
inheritor of both antique and Islamic civilisations. For that reason it
represents a blended and multidimensional identity. This chapter is
devoted to the concept of medical futility in Turkey from the point of
view of medical law and bioethics. Against this background, the healthcare system in Turkey, healthcare payment system, ethics in end-of-life
care in the country, medical futility concept in Turkey, relevant legislation, and the decision-making process are elaborated.

INTRODUCTION

Futility (futile medical care) is when a certain diagnosis or treatment is lacking beneficial results. The benefit referred to in this definition indicates benefits such as extending lifespan, reducing pain, and enabling comfort. Futile treatment can be considered if the intervention does not produce the desired physiological effect, the patient is going to die in the near future even if the intervention is carried out, there is a terminal condition etiologically and the planned intervention will not resolve the said condition, or the intervention does not help to increase the quality of life to the desired level (Kopelman 1995).

The basic conditions required to discuss medical futility in terms of bioethics are defined as a value judgement that falls on the thin line between useful and useless with a physical, psychological, or economic burden.

This article elaborates how futility, at a basic level, is perceived in Turkey, whether there are legal regulations in force regarding the subject, and how and by whom decisions are made in practice. First, this chapter explains the healthcare system and the ethical approach to death in Turkey in order to set a background regarding the subject.

THE HEALTHCARE SYSTEM IN TURKEY

Turkey is a country with a population of 72.5 million (a rural population ratio of 25.0%, an urban population ratio of 75.0%, a 0–14 aged population ratio of 26.3%, and a 65 and 65+ aged population ratio of 6.8%), a national income per person of 8,590 USD, and a per capita public and private health expenditure of 814 USD. Health-related figures illustrate that the life expectancy at birth is 73.6 (75.8 female, 71.4 male), the infant mortality rate is 17.0 (per 1,000 live births), there are 1,350 hospitals (847 state hospitals, 400 private hospitals), and the number of health personnel per 1,000 population is 0.89 physicians, 0.61 midwives, 0.98 nurses, and 0.28 dentists (T.C. Sağlık Bakanlığı 2010).

The history of the healthcare system in the Republic of Turkey can be analysed in three periods:

1) The Foundation and Institutionalisation Period (1923–1960): Health services were established for the first time, and spread nationwide.
2) The Socialisation Period (1961–1979): Health services were a fundamental task conducted by the government, with the understanding that health services were a "right."
3) The Liberal Period (1980–2010): A part of the health services' public nature was abandoned and privatised (Arda and Güvercin 2010).

Healthcare was among the priorities set by Mustafa Kemal Atatürk, the founder of the Republic of Turkey. This is why one of the first laws issued by the Turkish Grand National Assembly, founded on 23 April 1920, during the years of the Turkish War of Independence, was the law to establish the Ministry of Health. With this law, health services were accepted as a public service conducted by a ministry of the state. After founding a republic, the objective was to establish and organise health services in a country that wars had destroyed, spread the healthcare throughout the country, and institutionalise it. Health was important as it was the key to achieving sufficient manpower in terms of quality and quantity. During this period, almost 50 laws, still in force today, were adopted between 1923 and 1937 by Dr. Refik Saydam, the Minister of Health at the time. The primary objectives during this period were "central planning and exclusive structuring and organizing of the preventive and therapeutic health services as separate departments, filling the gap in health care personnel at the earliest possible time, and fighting against epidemic infectious diseases such as malaria, tuberculosis, trachoma, leprosy, and syphilis." Organisations providing health services were structured based on a vertical organisation model. The government built diagnosis and treatment centres and physicians were not allowed to have private practices. Primary healthcare services were popularised and health expenses were financed from the general budget. Treatment services provided to inpatients were also financed by public funds; however, it was adopted that these services were managed by local authorities. The purpose of the 10-Year Health Plan, established in 1946, was to integrate preventive and therapeutic health services, and spread them nationwide.

Law No. 224, adopted in 1961, initiated the "socialisation" period of health services; it was the biggest breakthrough in health, in the history of the country, up until that date. Healthy living was accepted as a birth right, and the government was appointed to do everything required within the context of this right. It was seen appropriate that the general budget financed healthcare services, and everybody should be included in the social security system. The health service should be based on the following characteristics: to comply with the principle of social justice and equality, to be population-based with priority given to preventive medicine, a team service with a referral system, public access, free of charge, as well as having collaboration with industries (Arda 2010).

The basic principles of socialisation comply with international regulations and views regarding health organisations. In order to establish public health at the international level, the socialisation law was established before the Alma-Ata Manifesto in 1978, which published and formulated Basic Health Services, the Health for Everyone in 2000 objectives in 1984, defined for Europe, and the Health 21 objectives, established in 1998, and played a significant role in establishing these principles. This law placed priority and importance on free service at health centres, integrated service for primary, secondary, and tertiary care, team services, population-based service, and preventive health services. This also set forth plans for mobile health services, ongoing training for personnel, community participation, inter-sector collaboration, a referral system, and all-day service.

Even though socialising healthcare services significantly improved the country's health index, such as reducing the infant mortality and maternal mortality rates, and preventing infectious diseases, it was not able to achieve the generalisation of nationwide healthcare services due to insufficient support and funds.

The military coup in Turkey in 1980 gave rise to a change in the nature of healthcare services, and the state started to abandon their fundamental duty in providing healthcare services. Health services started to lose their public nature, especially due to the effect of international financial organisations such as the World Bank and IMF, in the name of "reform in healthcare," and health services started to become a commodity offered to the market under free market conditions. During this period, in which general economic indicators deteriorated (for example, inflation reached 115%), the budget put aside for health decreased, public health investments nearly came to a standstill, and wages of healthcare staff were reduced. As a result, health services deteriorated in terms of quality and quantity, and the need arose for liberal adjustments in the health sector.

In line with privatisation activities, there was an increase in the share the private sector held within health services from 1990 onwards and the private sector grew even more with finance from public resources. In the 2000s, primary healthcare services started to be provided by "family practices," an examination-based system, instead of health centres which called the Health Transformation Programme. These circumstances indicated that preventive medicine was put on the back burner in health services, while therapeutic medicine took priority. Hospitals started to be converted into "businesses," and were privatised. The system was financed by premiums deducted from employees in the name of general health insurance. Public health expenses multiplied by four between 2002 and 2009 together with the transformation in the healthcare system. The main reason behind this increase was medical technology and drug costs. There were significant doubts as to whether or not the system could be sustained under such conditions.

After establishing the Republic of Turkey, the main objective was for the state to build a healthcare system and to generalise healthcare services throughout the country. The socialisation period in particular was a contemporary stage in which the aim was to make sure everybody's right to health was under constitutional guarantee and healthcare was accessible, free of charge, and high in quality. However, healthcare services started to be privatised during the liberal period. According to the Turkish Medical Association, this model is expensive and therapeutic, as opposed to preventive. In addition, the system does not take rural areas into consideration, causes competitiveness among doctors that is unethical, limits healthcare for chronic patients, disrupts the referral system, and hinders programmes such as vaccination and family planning. The Health Transformation Programme, which represents this era, continues to be questioned by the public, although it has become a significant part of practice, and made a place for itself (Arda 2010).

The Payment System in Healthcare

In Turkey, the term "general health insurance," stated in the Social Security and General Health Insurance Law (No. 5510, on 31 May 2006), refers to primarily protecting the health of individuals, and financing expenses incurred in the event that individuals are faced with health risks. In accordance with this law, benefiting from healthcare services and other rights offered by general health insurance is a right for those insured and their dependants, and the insurance organisation is obliged to generate the funds required to provide this service and right. The following are some of the healthcare services that are financed by the organisation:

a) Preventive healthcare services for individuals regardless of whether they are ill or not, and preventive healthcare services directed to prevent drug addiction that is harmful for individuals.

b) Health services and emergency health services required by inpatients or outpatients, clinical examinations deemed necessary by a doctor for diagnosis, laboratory investigations and other diagnostic methods, medical interventions and treatment conducted in accordance with diagnosis, patient follow-up and rehabilitation services, organ, tissue and stem cell transplants, and cell therapy.

c) For pregnant women, inpatient or outpatient, clinical examinations deemed necessary by a doctor for diagnosis, delivery, laboratory investigations, tests and other diagnostic methods, medical interventions and treatment conducted in accordance with diagnosis, patient follow-up, medical abortion, medical sterilisation, and emergency healthcare services.

d) For inpatients or outpatients, oral and dental examinations deemed necessary to diagnose oral and dental diseases, laboratory investigations, diagnosis-based medical interventions, and treatments.

e) A married woman with no child, or the spouse of a man with no child can benefit from assisted reproductive methods under their general health insurance. However, in order to qualify there are certain criteria that need to be met, and in the event that no other treatment method is possible, and the procedure is seen as the only option, assisted reproductive methods are offered, but the treatment is limited to two tries.

f)   Services related to the health services offered in accordance with the items stated above: blood and blood products, bone marrow, vaccinations, medications, orthesis, prosthesis, medical instruments, individual-specific medical devices, medical consumables, providing, installing and repairing medical consumables, including post-guarantee maintenance, repair and replacement services.

The following are health services that will not be financed by the insurance organisation:

a)   Any form of aesthetic-based health services that are not covered under health services conducted to reinstate physical integrity, and circumstances that arise due to occupational accidents, occupational illnesses or congenital reasons.
b)   Health services not licensed or approved by the Ministry of Health, and health services not accepted as medical health services by the Ministry of Health.
c)   For foreign citizens, health services for chronic diseases that are present before the date they become insured or a dependant of the insured, under general health insurance.

The following are cases in which a contribution will be requested from health services:

a)   Doctor and dentist examinations for outpatients.
b)   In vitro orthesis and prosthesis.
c)   Medication of outpatients.
d)   Financed health services for inpatients in accordance with patient groups determined by the organisation.

The following are cases in which a contribution will not be requested from health services:

a)   Health services provided for work accidents, occupational illnesses, and during military operation and manoeuvres.
b)   Health services provided in the event of disasters and war.

c) Family practice and preventive health services for individuals.
d) Health services for chronic diseases determined by the organisation, vital health services, and organ, tissue and stem cell transplants, provided that circumstances are documented with a health report.
e) Check-ups, etc. (Sosyal Sigortalar ve Genel Sağlık Sigortası Kanunu 2011).

ETHICS IN END-OF-LIFE CARE IN TURKEY

Nowadays, medical ethics are developing in a totally different direction from traditional approaches. This new direction tends to consider patient rights in a doctor-patient relationship, and initiate patient autonomy. In this respect, medical practice is dominated by an approach that takes patient wishes into account.

The most important point that comes up when the state of elderly patients are examined in the light of medical ethics is where elderly patients stand when distributing limited resources in daily medical practice. How can we assess geriatric care for the elderly population in terms of medical ethics? The question is when it is justified to use scarce resources at the end of life, for whom, and for what purpose. How we can discuss these issues but not discriminate against this group of patients?

One of the important issues touched upon regarding treatment costs in medical practice is treatment based solely on using high technology medicine. In this respect, whether or not it is necessary to provide elderly patients with medical interventions that are based on high technology and are extremely expensive has become a topic that is constantly questioned in terms of ethics. The pivotal point of this argument is whether or not it is more realistic to direct expensive treatment toward younger patients for satisfying results, or "waste" it on elderly patients, who do not have many years left to live. However, one should be aware that depriving patients of medical opportunities because of their age creates a slippery slope from which ill thoughts and approaches can arise.

In Turkey, there are no legal guidelines stating conditions under which treatment should be stopped, what the medical criteria are to determine such a condition, who should make such a decision, and the process they need to follow.

In terms of dealing with a request to end someone's life at the end of life in Turkey, euthanasia is not an option for example for a 60 year old with a brain tumour suffering severe pain, whose quality of life is accepted to be intolerable. Any intervention that directly affects an individual's life is not accepted by law.

For a different age group, for example a six year old with advanced cancer, there is nothing in the regulations that allows parents to withdraw treatment. In the event that parents refuse further treatment, doctors and family members can make a decision together. Every sort of intervention is carried out in order to treat a newborn that requires ventilation support for 23 weeks, without seeking family approval. It is very rare that a treatment team will discuss the request of a 13-year-old patient refusing treatment, when their family request that they are treated, and decide to discharge them (Platin 2007).

Another important issue when dealing with the aged population and ethics of end of life is the autonomy of elderly patients. From this point of view, we can say that elderly people are in a similar situation to that of special groups that have difficulties exercising their autonomy, such as children, psychiatric patients, and prisoners. This helps us to understand why elderly people are considered to be one of the special groups in therapeutic medicine, preventive medicine, and biomedical research. The Health for Everyone in the 21st Century objectives set by the World Health Organization in 2000 express that the health of the elderly has gained a different form of importance. Objectives under this heading are separated into two groups: "increasing the life expectancy of 65 year olds by 20% without disability," and "increasing the life expectancy of 80 year olds by at least 50% by enabling them to live in a healthy home environment, and giving them the opportunity to maintain their autonomy, self-respect, and place in society" (Öztürk and Arda 2007).

In dealing with end-of-life cases, autonomy is an important subject because in aged patients who are unable to exercise their right to autonomous decision making, due to the decrease in their competency, obtaining informed consent is always a concern while offering healthcare services.

Situations that have an adverse effect on autonomous decisions are a decrease in self-assessment ability, a slower reasoning capacity, displaying faults in decision making, and lack of knowledge in order to make a decision; all of these situations become an ethical concern in the decision-making process. As well as being a legal obligation, paying respect to an individual's autonomy is also an ethical obligation. Similarly, in the case of futile treatment, the patient's ability to contribute to the decision making regarding the course of treatment is very crucial. In order to define the importance of informed consent in practice, there is a need for an approach that takes into consideration its variable and restricted requirements.

The criterion used to make sure whether or not a patient can use her/his autonomy is the patient's competence in decision making. In terms of making decisions, individuals are either competent or incompetent. Having competence indicates that an individual can exercise their autonomy. Accordingly, the individual's competency is a must in order to talk about valid informed consent. The fundamental reason behind such a condition is that they need to have the capacity to understand the information provided, assess it, and make a suitable decision. The common approach is that the extent of competency is subject-specific as opposed to general. For example, the decision-making capacity of an elderly dementia patient, when asked whether they would like to be cared for at home or in a nursing home, can be evaluated based on whether or not they can differentiate between the two environments, and if they are aware of the conclusions that arise under both circumstances. The fact that competence can deteriorate over time should also be taken into consideration. It is common that the competence of elderly and dementia patients gradually deteriorates, hence competence evaluation should be repeated regularly.

Protecting the autonomy of incompetent patients and preventing them from losing their rights is seen as a doctor's ethical responsibility. In the event that medical opportunities cannot provide standard treatment, triage is a method actively used to resolve the issues. This method groups applicants as "likely to die, regardless of what care they receive," "likely to live, regardless of what care they receive," and "immediate care might make a positive difference in outcome." It is recommended that treatment should be offered to those under the last group. A different type of susceptibility is required to assess patients under such terms. Anti-ageism sets forth that it is unjust that people's lives are ended; the reasons it puts forward are that for those that want to live, the remaining years are precious, nobody deserves to die so long as they want to live, and there are those that have a longer life expectancy. The contradictory argument, the "justified time" argument, assumes that 70 years is a reasonable lifespan, and states that those that do not reach the age of 70 have been hard done by, and those that live past 70 are living on borrowed time. This argument sets forth that everyone should have the chance to reach the justified age, and those that have reached the justified age should give up their extra years for those that need it. Of course, both views have their limitations; the "justified time" argument can be valid in situations where medical opportunities are limited, but for all other situations, the anti-ageism argument is more suitable; individuals should not be treated with negative discrimination just because they are elderly.

Getting patients to articulate their requests regarding their future health while they still have their decision-making capacity is a form of practice that is becoming more common. In traditional communities, the method used most often is that the doctor offers recommendations from which the patient will benefit the most, and obtains the consent of the patient's family accordingly. In the event that patients have consented to donating their organs after death, the family also needs to consent for the organs to be donated. This reminds us of the concepts such as relatives, family, and family consent that have functions in different cultural structures. In Turkey, in end-of-life decision making, in the event of lack of consensus among the patient, family, and the physician, a resolution may be sought by approaching the ethics committee of the hospital.

MEDICAL FUTILITY: LEGISLATION AND THE DECISION-MAKING PROCESS

Ethical dilemmas are frequently experienced in intensive care units due to increased clinical opportunities in intensive care, and the fact that new technologies are used in intensive care units very frequently (Iyilikçi *et al.* 2004). Death-related issues are at the forefront in intensive care units, which is why ethical dilemmas are quite frequent. Some of the ethical dilemmas experienced are the futility or ineffectiveness of treatment, whether life support treatment should commence or not, whether ongoing life support treatment should continue or be stopped, and whether or not cardiopulmonary resuscitation should be conducted (Çobanoğlu and Algıer 2004).

In the case of medical futility, a physician may deprive the patient of treatment by withholding or withdrawing treatment against the will of the patient/representative because the treatment (requested) does not have any useful purpose. Therefore, in this situation, the concepts of professional integrity and patient autonomy clash and create an ethical dilemma (Ersoy 2003).

Even though there are numerous studies that have been conducted in many countries regarding practices of doctors when faced with death-related issues and do-not-resuscitate (DNR) orders, there are no reports in Turkey that investigate how doctors make death-related decisions, and whether or not social factors affect these decisions. However, regarding DNR orders, Iyilikçi *et al.* (2004) considered this and conducted a study that assessed the practice of Turkish anaesthesiologists under such circumstances. In the study, 65.9% of participants stated that they execute written and verbal DNR orders. These decisions are mainly based on discussions with the other physicians (82.7%) before being made; discussion with the family, or with the patient, or the ethics committee seems not to be the preferred way in daily practice. Only 6% of DNR instructions are written, the remaining 94% are verbal. The majority of DNR requests in North European countries are written, and the fact that DNR requests in Turkey are mostly verbal illustrates how the topic is unrelated to legal rights and obligations, or other practical views. According to responses which participating doctors gave to a case presented by researchers, it was concluded that Turkish doctors prefer to continue, or limit, treatment instead of withdrawing treatment or giving the patient painkillers in situations where treatment should not be initiated or withdrawn. While most European doctors believe that withholding or withdrawing life support are primarily biomedical and ethical issues, where the doctor should make the decision, doctors in Turkey inform families that their patient has no chance of recovery, but families insist that the patient should be provided with full life support (Iyilikçi *et al.* 2004).

A study, conducted to understand the international difference in decisions made in intensive care units regarding death, concluded that DNR requests differentiated according to geography; while those participating from Australia, Canada, the USA, and Northern and Central European countries gave written DNR instructions, those participating from Turkey, Southern Europe, and Brazil preferred to give DNR instructions verbally. Among the obtained results was the fact that participants from Turkey and Japan frequently chose to sustain full life support together with choosing aggressive treatment in comparison to other participating countries (Yaguchi et al. 2005).

A study, conducted to prevent potential conflicts caused when determining and resolving ethical issues perceived by doctors and nurses working in intensive care in Turkey, concluded that the most common ethical issue which doctors and nurses working in intensive care face is death-related decision making. Death-related decisions made in intensive care are decisions as to whether the death of the patients should be delayed or whether it should be speeded up. This study set forth ethical issues, such as euthanasia, refusing treatment, futile treatment, brain death, DNR decisions, commodification, organ donation, and autonomy, under the basic category of death-related decision making (Çobanoğlu and Algıer 2004). Passive euthanasia was analysed in the context of not providing or withdrawing treatment. In this study, a significant portion of doctors (68.4%) reported that they considered futile treatment as an ethical issue, while nurses made no comment. On the other hand, while physical restraints were a major issue for nurses, doctors made no comment. This proved that doctors and nurses defined ethical issues based on their area of responsibility due to the nature of their professional roles. The fact that doctors are more susceptible regarding whether or not treatment is futile can be interpreted as part of their role or physician paternalism.

In 2005, Akpinar et al. (2009) conducted a study regarding death-related decisions making by nurses working in paediatric intensive care. The study concluded that 65% of nurses could not accept not initiating pointless (futile) treatment, and 60% of nurses could not accept withdrawing treatment. Sixty-eight percent of nurses accepted that intravenous feeding should continue regardless of the consequences. In terms of futile treatment, nurses had a tendency to leave the decision to parents, or act in a paternalistic way. According to study results, authors reported that nurses ruled out their death-related ethical responsibilities, and concluded that nurses working in intensive care units in Turkey definitely require training about the principle of doing no harm, the principle of justice, and death-related ethical issues such as the pointlessness or futility of treatment. In addition, authors reported that cultural values directly affected the habits of healthcare staff, and how they were well-established. However, they suggested that these habits could be changed by providing training about death-related ethical issues, especially on the subject of medical futility in intensive care (Akpinar *et al.* 2009).

There are still no distinctive death-related laws or ethical legal regulations in Turkey. For example, there are no legal examples in Turkey defining whether or not a doctor has the authority to make death-related decisions, to limit or withdraw support from terminal or seriously ill patients (Iyilikçi *et al.* 2004).

Ersoy (2003) argues that a doctor has the right to refuse conducting a medically futile intervention based on Article 6 of the Patient Rights Act of 1998, which relates to medical futility and suggests that in order for medical resources to be distributed justly it should be on a need basis. The relevant article of the Patient Rights Act is Article 6, which states:

> "The patient has the right to benefit from health services in accordance with their needs, including preventive health services and activities related to encouraging healthy living within the framework of justice and equity rights. This right also includes the obligation all healthcare organisations, institutions, and healthcare staff have towards complying with justice and equality principles (Hasta Hakları Yönetmeliği 2009)."

MEDICAL FUTILITY AND EUTHANASIA

A case narrative: "In some cases you can "feel the hurt" with the patient. A Stage IV small cell lung cancer patient was begging for help to die because of the severe shortness of breath. None of the sedative drugs could sedate her. The situation was discussed with the family. The possibility that the patient could not be awakened when put to sleep was discussed with the family. Everyone agreed with this possibility since no one could any longer tolerate the patient's begging and crying. IV infusion of one ampoule of midazolam was started. An hour later the patient had died. This was an inevitable end for the patient. The patient was comfortable. Patients have the right to die also. Therefore law changes are needed these concepts should be considered within the understanding of treatment (Platin 2007)."

The term "euthanasia" comes from Latin, meaning "good death." Even though it has been disguised in many different shapes and forms since ancient times, euthanasia is an important subject that continues to be scrutinised in ethical debates. Euthanasia is grouped under three different categories: doctor's order, patient's request, and the nature of the procedure. Euthanasia upon patient request is divided into three groups: voluntary euthanasia, non-voluntary euthanasia, and involuntary euthanasia. A granted right creates grounds for everyone that could benefit from exercising that right. There are question marks as to whether or not euthanasia is a right because there are several situations in medicine in which the patient's consent cannot be obtained. Subject-related examples in local regulations show that euthanasia is not seen as a patient right in Turkey. However, this situation does not eliminate ethical issues related to the subject.

Euthanasia is defined as passive or active, depending on the role the doctor plays during the process. Euthanasia can be considered an action against medicine, an occupation based entirely on "life" and "keeping the patient alive." This heading, which is a sore discussion spot for medicine, articulates arguments such as "even if we approve euthanasia under certain circumstances, this does not make us executioners," "active euthanasia cannot be something a doctor does, when their only task during death sentences is documenting the death," and "medicine saves the lives of individuals that have attempted suicide, and for the sake of internal consistence, medicine should protest against euthanasia." Some of the questions forming the discussion are as follows: Are there circumstances where medicine can justify "turning a blind eye," in situations where nothing else can be done for a patient, and "respect for life" an occupational principle? If doctors take on such a "task" will it disrupt the doctor-patient relationship which is based on trust?

In Turkey, on one hand, decision making about futile treatment is a sample of inadequate discussion; on the other hand, euthanasia and assisted suicide are strictly forbidden. Therefore, it is possible to sustain medical treatment and support in applications under every condition. A doctor that does not intervene to stop a suicide attempt may be perceived as assisting suicide. There are examples where such doctor attitudes, which take into consideration patient autonomy, are deemed illegal; however, subject-related ethical discussions are still considered insufficient (Arda 2002).

For example, if an individual has an accident at a young age and is left paraplegic, and he decides that he cannot live like that, and want to exercise his right to euthanasia, there is no place for such a request in Turkish medical law. There is no basis available that will take such a request into consideration. It is illegal to withdraw treatment, even if this patient becomes quadriplegic, is connected to a ventilator, and adamantly requests to be unplugged from the ventilator. Withdrawing treatment is not defined in medical regulations, and is not a part of general practice. However, under circumstances where the cost of treatment is highly expensive, relatives of the patient may be asked to take their patient home; this is accepted as a form of passive euthanasia. Bearing in mind that situations in which withdrawing or withholding life support is confused with passive euthanasia. In Turkey, euthanasia is an action that is generally considered illegal by law. According to Turkish Criminal Law No. 5237 (Türk Ceza Kanunu 2010), euthanasia falls under "manslaughter in the first degree."

The clearest clause regarding euthanasia is stated in the Patient Rights Act 1998. Article 13 of the Act, titled "Euthanasia Prohibition," says that "Under no circumstances can any individual abandon the right to live, whether by medical necessities, or in any other manner whatsoever. Nobody's life can be ended, upon request of the individual, or upon the request of another person" (Hasta Hakları Yönetmeliği 2009).

In terms of limiting or withdrawing life support, doctors in Turkey are obliged to comply with the Medical Deontology Regulation 1960 (Tıbbi Deontoloji Nizamnamesi 2009), in which Article 13 states it is not possible to conduct a procedure that will reduce the physical endurance of the patient, and Article 14 states that doctors are obliged to display due diligence required by a patient's condition.

Article 13/3 reads: "Doctors and dentists cannot conduct any actions, without diagnosis, treatment, or preventive purposes, which will reduce the mental or physical endurance of a patient upon request by the patient, or any other reasons." In this regard Article 14/1 emphasises that "Doctors and dentists will display the due diligence required in accordance with patient circumstances. They are obliged to reduce or put a stop to the pain endured, even in situations where it is impossible to protect the life and health of the patient."

CONCLUSION

Elderly patients suffering from chronic, progressive, and possibly terminal illnesses have a hope of getting better, and have expectations and rights to receiving treatment that is honourable as opposed to treatable. The due diligence that medicine is obliged to display is without a question also valid for elderly patients.

Bearing in mind that relatives of patients actively contribute to the process of decision making, the extent of doctor-patient relationships has expanded, and shared responsibility and decision making regarding the patient is getting more attention. However, doctors play a significant role in resolving issues faced during this process by making constructive and functional recommendations and it is obvious that doctors should display the required due diligence at this point. It can be argued that a doctor able to distinguish between treatment and care applications, achieve team work coordination, and provide the patient with compassion and attention in a humane approach during the diagnosis, treatment, and follow-up process, has the correct attitude in dealing with medical futility.

In the event that a patient in Turkey is thought to be receiving treatment that is medically futile, there is no law that allows treatment withdrawal. Euthanasia is classified as a crime by the Constitution in Turkey. However, based on daily practice, it is possible to state that passive euthanasia is exercised in certain cases.

It is possible to indicate that death-related discussions are extremely limited in the world of medicine in Turkey, and the subject is not touched upon enough during medical school. In fact, the same can be said for specialist physicians regarding their own education. In daily medical practice two different situations are mostly seen. One is where an accurate brain-dead diagnosis is made and after that the patient is taken off life support and artificial feeding procedures. The other one is where relatives of patients request treatment to be withdrawn and the patient discharged. Regardless of the differences, both situations have difficulties to struggle with and seems to be similar practices. On the one hand is the weight of making an irreversible decision in terms of the decision maker, and on the other hand the implications of making such decisions — being given various labels directed at the occupational identity, and reducing/damaging the trust of doctor-patient relationships. The serious issues regarding the professional role of physicians are providing treatment directed at saving the lives of patients that are not competent to make decisions, the possible benefits or whether such treatments are necessary or futile, the attitudes displayed by relatives of patients regarding the subject, and the ethical responsibility of delaying the death of an individual who is in pain due to the availability of technology. Therefore, it is necessary to address how far the effort to "insist on keeping the patient alive at all cost" ignores patient autonomy, and whether or not "a right to die" exists based on participation. We conclude that more empirical surveys to document public and professional attitudes towards end-of-life decision making in general and medical futility in particular are crucial for the healthcare system in Turkey.

REFERENCES

Akpinar A, Ozcan Senses M, and Aydin Er R. 2009. Attitudes to end-of-life decisions in paediatric intensive care. *Nursing Ethics* 16: 83–92.

Arda B. 2002. How should physicians approach a hunger strike? *Bulletin of Medical Ethics* 181: 13–18.

Arda B. 2010. Turkey's health system. Oral presentation in workshop, 18th World Congress for Medical Law, Zagreb, Croatia, August 8–12.

Arda B and Güvercin CH. 2010. Historical development of the Turkish Health System. Poster presentation in 18th World Congress for Medical Law, Zagreb, Croatia, August 8–12.

Çobanoğlu N and Algıer L. 2004. A qualitative analysis of ethical problems experienced by physicians and nurses in intensive care units in Turkey. *Nursing Ethics* 11: 444–458.

Ersoy N. 2003. Yaşamın sonuyla ilgili etik konular: I [Ethical issues related to end-of-life: I]. In: A Demirhan Erdemir, O Öncel Ö, and Ş Aksoy, eds. *Çağdaş Tıp Etiği* (Contemporary medical ethics). Istanbul: Nobel Tıp Kitabevleri, pp. 328–357 (in Turkish).

Hasta Hakları Yönetmeliği (Patient Rights Act). Resmi Gazete (Official Gazette), Tarihi, August 1, 1998, Sayısı, No: 23420. Available at: http://www.mevzuat. gov.tr/Metin.Aspx?MevzuatKod=7.5.4847&MevzuatIliski=0&sourceXmlSe arch=Hasta hakları (in Turkish) [Accessed June 4, 2012].

Iyilikçi L, Erbayraktar S, Gökmen N, Ellidokuz H, Kara HC, and Günerli A. 2004. Practices of anaesthesiologists with regard to withholding and withdrawal of life support from the critically ill in Turkey. *Acta Anaesthesiologica Scandinavica* 48: 457–462.

Kopelman LM. 1995. Conceptual and moral disputes about futile and useful treatments. *Journal of Medicine and Philosophy* 20: 109–121.

Öztürk H and Arda B. 2007. Yaşlılık ve etik sorunlar (Geriatrics and ethical problems). In: Y Gökçe-Kutsal, ed. *Temel Geriatri* (Basic geriatrics). Ankara: Güneş Tıp Kitabevleri, pp. 371–377 (in Turkish).

Platin N. 2007. Personal interview, Ankara, January 15.

Sosyal Sigortalar ve Genel Sağlık Sigortası Kanunu (Social Insurance and General Health Insurance Law) (in Turkish). Available at: http://www.sgk. gov.tr/wps/wcm/connect/018b41a5–8f47–4034-a170–14eb7 [Accessed June 4, 2012].

TC Sağlık Bakanlığı (The Ministry of Health). Available at: http://www.saglik. gov.tr (in Turkish) [Accessed March 1, 2011].

Tıbbi Deontoloji Nizamnamesi (Medical Deontology Regulations). Resmi Gazete (Official Gazette) Tarihi, February 19, 1960, Sayısı NO: 10436. (in Turkish). Available at: http://www.mevzuat.gov.tr/Tuzukler.aspx [Accessed June 4, 2012].

Türk Ceza Kanunu. Kanun No: 5237 (Turkish Criminal Law). Available at: http:// www.mevzuat.gov.tr/Kanunlar.aspx (in Turkish) [Accessed June 4, 2012].

Yaguchi A, Truog RD, Curtis R *et al.* 2005. International differences in end-of-life attitudes in the intensive care unit. *Archives of Internal Medicine* 165: 1970–1975.

CHAPTER TWELVE

MEDICAL FUTILITY IN THE UNITED ARAB EMIRATES

Said Abuhasna and Ali Abdulkareem Al Obaidli

SUMMARY

This chapter presents the approach to medical futility in the United Arab Emirates (UAE) and the surrounding region, by explaining the health-care system, decision making regarding end-of-life issues in general and medical futility in particular, as well as related laws and guidelines.

The UAE has a universal healthcare system, which provides access to healthcare for all of its citizens. Unlike in Western societies, limited research has been conducted on the end-of-life issues in the UAE. With the expansion of the local population and with the growing numbers of practicing Emirati physicians, discussions about end-of-life care has been increasing. Medical symposiums and conferences have been held around the country addressing the need for awareness among professionals and patients about this subject and hospitals have started offering palliative care for terminally ill patients. However, in the UAE, limiting medical treatment deemed futile is a new concept with no legal definition. The most acceptable form in dealing with medical futility is to limit further medical interventions. Formulating a national policy based on physicians' attitudes and the perceptions of patients and families is necessary to clarify the legal position on end-of-life decisions in general and medical futility in particular.

INTRODUCTION

The Gulf Cooperation Council (GCC), is composed of six countries: the United Arab Emirates (UAE), the Kingdom of Saudi Arabia, Oman, Kuwait, Qatar and the Kingdom of Bahrain. They share the same religion, culture and customs.

These countries are an integral part of the wider Arab region. They are deeply rooted in Arab culture and history, and Islam represented by the Qur'an and Hadith is the fabric of this society. The countries of the GCC are located on or near the Arabian Peninsula that comprises an area of 2,500,000 km² and a population of approximately 42 million according to a 2012 census. The unified economic agreement between these countries was signed on November 11, 1981, in Abu Dhabi, the capital of the UAE.

The main resource of the Gulf Cooperation Council countries is oil. However, these countries have begun an aggressive policy of reforms and structural changes with the aim of diversifying their economies through building strong industrial-based economies as well as providing the necessary infrastructure to be tourist destinations and/or service and financial hubs as well as centers for trade and transit between Asia and Europe. All GCC states have experienced unprecedented socioeconomic transformation that has led to higher standards of living, stable currencies and low inflation rates. The local populations of the GCC countries are generally small and therefore a high proportion of the work force consists of expatriates from other countries. The prevailing political and social system of these states is mostly conservative and tribal in nature with strong family and tribal ties. One common theme that bonds all GCC countries is the religion of Islam and the Shari'a law. In this chapter, we will give the UAE as an example to discuss medical futility and end-of-life issues because what applies to the UAE is likely to apply to the rest of the GCC countries.

Historically, the UAE was established by unification of seven emirates. The UAE became a fully independent country on December 2, 1971. While the UAE has worked to strengthen its federal institutions since achieving independence, each of the seven emirates still maintains substantial autonomy. Currently the population of the UAE is close to 8.9 million residents in 2012, less than 15% of which are local citizens. The balance of the population is made up of aliens who reside in the UAE. Greater than one third of this population is from the Indian sub-continent and South-east Asia, while a significant number are from Europe and North Africa. The majority of Emirati citizens are Muslims with an average life expectancy of 74.3 years (UAE National Bureau of Statistics 2010).

The UAE has made significant progress in its healthcare system over the past 41 years. The healthcare sector continues to undergo major transformations to ensure that it is well integrated in order to meet international healthcare standards (Blair and Sharif 2012). Educational standards are rising rapidly in the UAE. Citizens and temporary residents have taken advantage of higher education facilities throughout the country. Many foreign institutions, including American, British and Australian universities, have established branches in the UAE. A developing country such as the UAE, which has taken substantial strides in its healthcare system and delivery, should be prepared to address end-of-life issues.

THE HEALTHCARE SYSTEM IN THE UAE AND OTHER GCC COUNTRIES

The GCC governments have made substantial investments in healthcare infrastructure during the past 25 years, building hospitals and clinics. They have promoted a more modern approach to tackling infectious diseases, such as malaria and measles that were once rampant in the region. Although differences exist from country to country, the overall improvement has been impressive. The average life expectancy rose from 60.5 years in 1978 to 73 years in 2004; during the same period, infant mortality fell from 69 deaths per 1,000 live births to 18. The average crude birth rate is 18.4% and crude death rate is 2.9%. Those below 15 years old make up 19.7% of the total population, while those greater than 65 years of age comprise only 1.6% of the population.

Healthcare demand and spending are rising sharply in the GCC countries. Policy makers would like to see the private sector play a greater role in their healthcare systems, in both the delivery of healthcare to the population and the financing of healthcare. To promote the private sector's involvement, the GCC governments must make major regulatory and policy changes and, above all, use public funds to reimburse nationals for the private healthcare services they consume, and define and enforce a single set of quality standards for both public and private healthcare delivery systems. The GCC countries had universal free healthcare coverage extending to all citizens for the past years until recently when the pattern of healthcare financing changed in an effort to optimize access to healthcare and the quality of healthcare, particularly following the introduction of healthcare insurance systems. The UAE started gradually to implement the mandatory health insurance requirement. This process started faster in some emirates with others following in their footsteps.

There are different classes of health insurance with subsidized basic plans for low-income people; however, others have enhanced plans.

ETHICS IN END-OF-LIFE ISSUES IN THE UAE

Death has become a process rather than an event. It no longer occurs in the home but in a medical institution. Sir William Osler once said, "Even the face of healthcare has changed, the fundamental nature of the practice of medicine is still the science of uncertainty and the art of probability." Physicians practicing in the West are encouraged to discuss advance directives with their terminally ill patients and their patients' families, especially when the prognosis is poor. It is because the concept of respect of patient autonomy and choice is accepted and implied that futility of care needs to be balanced with performing the maximum effort to save patients' lives.

From an Islamic perspective, there are no clear guidelines on end-of-life care for a Muslim patient. The first Arab Muslim country that started applying end-of-life care guidelines was the Kingdom of Saudi Arabia despite a lack of legal policy, and with the support of Islamic scholars' fatwas. In Arab Muslim countries, the relationship between patient and physician is one of traditional paternalism, based on the principles of goodness and kindness. This is no different from Christianity, whose adherents are directed to do good to others in a spirit of love and kindness (Damghi et al. 2011).

The Shari'a law, which governs the societies in Arab and Muslim countries, is based on the Holy Qur'an, the text believed by Muslims to be the direct word of God. The second is the Sunnah, the examples in words or deeds of the Prophet Muhammad, that is often incorporated into Islamic laws, and the third is the Ijtihad, the law of deductive logic.

In Islamic Shari'a, the definition of death has been accepted as when either of the two following signs is noted: First, when the heartbeat and breathing stop completely and the doctors believe that they cannot be restarted. Second, when all the functions of the brain have ceased, experienced doctors and specialists confirm that this is irreversible and the brain (as a whole) has started to disintegrate (Administration of Islamic Research and Ifta 1988). Most Islamic countries have endorsed these definitions. In the UAE both the General Authority of Islamic Affairs and Endowments (Awqaf) and the Ministry of Justice recently endorsed these definitions of death as well.

From the Islamic scholars' perspective, there is a consensus that end-of-life issues and even withdrawal of ventilatory support is acceptable in cases that meet the definition of death or in cases where three physicians have determined that the patient is clinically dead (Damghi *et al.* 2011). This has enabled physicians in Saudi Arabia, for example, to implement their own end-of-life decisions without necessarily securing consent from the family.

The UAE has a diverse group of practicing physicians from all over the world. These physicians are from different countries and origins — the Middle East countries, the USA, Europe, Australia and African countries. With the growing number of practicing local Emirati physicians, the end-of-life concept has been more in discussion than ever before. Symposiums and conferences have been held addressing the need for awareness about end-of-life issues. Some hospitals have started offering palliative care for terminally ill patients. There is a growing understanding in the health ministry of the UAE for the need to have a federal policy on dealing with terminally ill patients.

MEDICAL FUTILITY IN THE UAE: WHO MAKES THE DECISION?

Medical futility refers to interventions that are unlikely to produce significant benefits for the patient. In the UAE, most of the physicians and other healthcare providers agree with the international standard definitions, particularly when supported by Islamic endorsement. This has paved the way for the implementation of deceased organ transplantation programs similar to those in most other Islamic countries.

As Islam teaches, everyone will face death, and the manner in which we die is of great individual importance. Comforting the dying is a must. Although guidelines for healthcare providers in delivering comfort care to the dying patient will be invaluable to staff covering end-of-life situations and spare the patient from futile interventions, there is a lack of such guidelines in the UAE. These guidelines would be helpful in explaining who makes the decision for resuscitation, how the decision is made, and the role of patients and their families in the decision making. With the development of widely accepted Islamic guidelines on futile care as practiced in Saudi Arabia, UAE physicians may follow such guidelines for treating terminally ill patients.

There is a growing understanding about the futility of care for terminally ill patients in clinical settings and the concept of palliative care is gaining momentum in the UAE as well as the rest of the Islamic countries. With the increasing number of patients with terminal diseases and the limited intensive care resources in the UAE, the time may be right for addressing end-of-life care issues with the involvement of healthcare policy makers, as it has been practiced in the West and some other Islamic countries which adopted the guidelines. For the time being, an available resource for physicians would be experiences or guidelines from Western countries as well as other Islamic countries in the care of terminally ill patients if such guidelines exist. Among physicians, critical care physicians are best suited to address this issue. We gauged these assumptions in a survey that we recently conducted, which included a questionnaire related to the management of terminally ill patients, which was sent electronically to the members of the Pan-Arab Critical Care Physicians. The questionnaire was to compare the opinions of physicians who were educated in the West versus the ones educated in non-Western countries (Abuhasna *et al.* 2009). We found that all physicians agreed on having guidelines to deal with end-of-life care issues. There was no statistically significant difference between the two groups with regard to rendering futile care to patients.

Although technology exists to sustain vital functions of almost any patient in an intensive care setting, not every patient is a candidate for the initiation and maintenance of life support measures.

Many critical care physicians encounter the situation of futility of care for terminally ill patients and the need to "bring the family on board" with realistic expectations about the prognosis. A lack of clear understanding about the prognosis of terminal illnesses leads families in the UAE to persist with futile treatments, which raises many ethical and practical questions. Optimal education of patients and their families often resolve these difficult situations for patients, families and their caregivers.

On the issue of resuscitation of terminally ill patients in Islamic bioethics, the following has been cited from the Qur'an (39:42): "There are times when human beings need to recognize their own limits and entrust nature to take its own course."

The Prophet (SAW) said while addressing the person whose funeral rites he was reading, "How fortunate you are that you died while you were not afflicted with illness" (Sahih Bukhari).

At several Islamic Jurist Committee meetings held in Mecca and Jeddah, and at the 3rd International Conference of Islamic Jurists in Amman in 1986, end-of-life issues were discussed in detail. At the meeting in Amman, Muslim jurists from different schools ruled that once invasive treatment has been intensified to save the life of a patient, life-saving equipment cannot be turned off unless the physicians are certain about the inevitability of death (Islamic Jurists 1990).

In many cultures, families and physicians are readily prepared to disclose the truth regarding the patient's illness. The ethics of a number of Asian and Eastern countries such as the UAE requires fatal diagnoses and bad prognoses to be disclosed to a family member.

However, the truth is often concealed for fear that it will extinguish the patient's hope, leading to despondence, physical suffering and mental anguish (Mobeireek et al. 2008). Disclosing the truth is therefore regulated by the prevailing concern for patient beneficence.

The right to refuse medical treatment is well established in medicine and law. When cases arose asserting that a patient had the right to be free of unwanted medical interventions, the right was readily recognized and clearly affirmed. In the UAE, with Arab and Muslim cultures, illness is a shared family affair. Consequently, decision making is family centered and beneficence and non-maleficence play a dominant role in their ethical model, in contrast to patient autonomy in Western cultures.

In the UAE and the majority of Arab nations, religious and cultural issues often play a more vital role in decision making by families and physicians than economic considerations.

In Saudi Arabia, for example, futile treatment is advocated and often requested by the patient's family (Albar 1996). This is the same in the UAE; however, this is a subject of great dispute, even among Islamic scholars. Some actively do not advocate treatment if it is to merely prolong the final stages of life (death). Moreover, they stress that delaying death with futile treatment is unacceptable in Islam; the Qur'an encourages the recognition of one's own limits. Islamic law, therefore, permits the withdrawal or withholding of futile or disproportionate treatment when consent is obtained from a family member, allowing death to take its natural course. Of importance is a study in Lebanon looking at withholding and withdrawing treatment in an intensive care unit, which highlighted concerns that the shift of focus to palliative care was taking place inappropriately late in the course of the patient's illness (Sachedina 2005). There is thus recognition that delaying the inevitable death of a patient is neither in the patient's nor in the public's best interests. According to Islam, the physician needs to be certain of the inevitability of the impending death, and if not, then life should be sustained. The futility of end-of-life treatment, however, can be difficult to define. This is due to several factors such as the effect on quality and length of life, emotional costs, financial costs and the likelihood of success. In Islamic culture, withholding therapy seems to be a more acceptable mode than limiting futile treatment when based on the physician's advice and consensus of family members (Takrouri and Halwani 2008; Fatwa No. 115104).

In fact, physicians in the UAE are often reluctant to discuss the subject of end-of-life care with patients or their family members out of the belief that it will not be accepted. They fear that talking about such issues may cause a loss of trust in the physician (Da Costa *et al.* 2002).

In result, a lack of discussion about futile care increases the length of stay in the intensive care unit as well as to a significant extent the number of survivors in a permanent vegetative state, which has led to a shortage of intensive care beds in the recent past. However, this approach is fading away and currently physicians understand the importance of approaching Emirati families to discuss end-of-life care issues in general and futile treatment in particular.

Currently, in a large hospital in Abu Dhabi, which has a palliative care program, the idea of comfort care or limiting futile treatment is very well received by the family members of patients who are admitted to the ICU. In this model, care conferences led by a senior member of the team are held to discuss the course of the patient's illness and issues related to futility of care and end-of-life care. Once a decision is made about the end-of-life care plan, the senior member of the team will communicate this to the rest of the team, including the nurses and ancillary staff. In our own survey mentioned earlier, the results are consistent with those of Da Costa et al. (2002). Subsequently, we surveyed 210 family members who are considered the proxy decision makers for the patients and we asked them if they would make a decision to limit the therapy for their loved one. The majority (about 75%) were reluctant to make such a decision and preferred to have the physician make the decision. A significant number of proxy decision makers asked the physician what he/she would do if it were their own family member (Abuhasna et al. 2009). Takrouri and Halwani recently published their study about end-of-life care from an Islamic point of view. They concluded that the consensus on this question is still evolving in the Islamic communities and that the Islamic verdicts, judicial opinions, or fatwas, were indicating that the decision of medical futility was to be decided by competent physicians involved in the care of the particular patient (Takrouri and Halwani 2008).

In our survey, which was conducted in the UAE, withholding treatment was the preferred method of end-of-life care interventions. The process of withholding the patient's life support frequently involves several discussions with the family as treatment goals are re-addressed when the probability of survival declines. Once the decision is made not to escalate therapy, the goal of treatment changes from attempts at curing to providing comfort measures. Therefore, the use of aggressive interventions, including dialysis, inotropic support and mechanical ventilation, would have to be justified in terms of providing comfort care to the patient.

In terms of decision making for an unconscious patient, in Western societies, advance directives are a well-known concept. The advance directive is synonymous with *Al Wasiya* in Arabic. However, the importance of Al Wasiya has been emphasized in the Qur'an: "Prescribed for you when death approaches [any] one of you if he leaves wealth [is that he should make] a bequest for the parents and near relatives according to what is acceptable — a duty upon the righteous" (2:180). This is also reiterated by the Prophet (PUH) who said, "It is not right for any Muslim who has something to be given as a bequest to spend two nights without writing a will about it," (narrated by Ibn Umar, may Allah be pleased with him) in Al-Bukhari and Muslim.

In the Western countries when patients lose their mental capacity but had indicated in an advance directive that they did not want life-prolonging procedures, courts have ruled that their advance wishes should be followed (Sprung *et al.* 2003). However, this is not the case in the United Arab Emirates.

When it comes to end-of-life care decision making, it appears to be influenced more by culture than religion. Another issue that is probably most influential in end-of-life decision making in this region is the structure of the family. The Emirati family is built on respect of the elder. The eldest makes the decision in the family and it usually goes in the following descending order: The father, the eldest son, followed by the second and third sons. If none of these are available, the grandfather on the father's side would be the sole decision maker in such a situation in the clinical setting for end-of-life care. This may be interpreted as the proxy decision maker in an advance directive. Many proxies feel uncomfortable in deciding to forgo life-prolonging interventions because they see themselves as deciding between life and death for another person. Since currently there are no laws on terminal care or advance directives, the physician must turn to the proxy and discuss the terminal illness care and be prepared to provide advice and guidance to the proxy.

One study which included 220 patients in an intensive care unit of a government hospital in the UAE aimed to assess if the (proxy) decision maker in the family was willing to sign consent to withdraw care for their dying family member. Among the respondents, 75% of the decision makers refused to sign consent to withdraw medical support for their loved ones. When asked about their reasoning for not signing such consent, 81% of them stated that "they felt guilty". So making the decision to withdraw treatment for the patient in the UAE is a process that places the heaviest burden on the attending physician (consultant) caring for the patient.

Attitudes of Healthcare Providers and the Public towards Medical Futility

End-of-life care decision making is in fact a religiously, emotionally and politically charged issue. Islam teaches us that everyone will face death, and the way an individual dies is of great importance. A survey has been recently conducted by our group to evaluate the attitudes of healthcare providers in the UAE towards end-of-life issues in dying, terminally ill patients. The questionnaire was formulated by our critical care team that deals with end-of-life care issues and was sent to all members of the Pan-Arab Society of Intensive Care Medicine. Most of the respondents were Muslim consultants with a Western training background. One question asked for their opinion on whether religion played a significant role in making decisions for a terminally ill patient. The majority of the respondents replied that religion played a major role in making end-of-life care decisions. Most of the intensivists worked in hospitals in which there were no end-of-life care guidelines. The lack of guidelines led to a variety of practices and approaches to handle the end-of-life issue in terminally ill patients. When presented with three futile case scenarios — a patient in a permanent vegetative state, a patient with renal carcinoma with metastasis, and a comatose patient with massive pulmonary embolism and multiple cerebral infarcts on a ventilator — the respondents preferred not to provide aggressive therapies (Abuhasna *et al.* 2009). In regard to the question about euthanasia, the majority of the respondents rejected it as it was totally unacceptable in Middle Eastern culture. Almost half of the respondents wanted physicians to have the ultimate authority in end-of-life care decision making. Physicians were equally split on overriding the wishes of the family on the no-code decision.

THE LINK BETWEEN MEDICAL FUTILITY AND EUTHANASIA

Euthanasia, derived from the Greek term for "good death", refers to the intentional hastening of death of a patient by a physician with the intent of alleviating suffering. Euthanasia may be carried out by administering medications to cause death or by withdrawing treatment that is essential to keep the patient alive. Pain relief and sedation do not fall within the scope of euthanasia. The issue of euthanasia has long been a matter of debate in medical, social, legal and religious domains. Islam categorically forbids all forms of suicide, and any action that may assist the person or patient to kill himself or herself is forbidden. Islam firmly upholds the sanctity of human life. The Qur'an says: "And do not take life — which God has made sacred — except for just cause" (17:33). In another passage, God says that someone taking an innocent life would be as if he had killed all humankind. It is not permitted for a Muslim to plan or choose the time of his own death in advance. There is a saying in which the Prophet Muhammad (PUH) refuses to bless the body of a person who had committed suicide. If, for example, someone is suffering from advanced cancer, but the person is not at risk of imminent death, Islam would prohibit the person from prematurely ending his or her life. Although euthanasia is not permitted, if a patient is critically ill, on life support and there is no hope for meaningful recovery, Islamic law would allow the patient's family to request the physician not to provide medical care and let nature take its course. This is not "mercy killing", but an acceptance of the fact that in this instance, medical treatment is only serving to prolong the dying process.

CONCLUSION

The United Arab Emirates is an Arab and Muslim country, which follows Islamic rules when it comes to the sanctity of life, medical care and end-of-life care. In Islamic ethics, family and community are intrinsically linked with each individual's well-being and illness is a shared family event rather than an individual issue. The family provides a source of strength, hope and connectedness to others. Accordingly, the principle of autonomy does not bear the same weight as it does in many Western cultures and thus the family is the locus of the decision-making process, especially when it comes to end-of-life care. Equally, in the United Arab Emirates, information regarding a patient's illness belongs to the family, who then may use the information in the best interests of the patient. Physicians, consequently, respect the autonomy of the family as a unit.

While death by the neurological criteria of brain death has become an accepted standard for pronouncing a patient dead in the Western countries, it has not yet received wide acceptance in the UAE, partly for cultural and religious reasons. Most family members still do not accept that their brain-dead loved one is in fact dead. In practice, allowing adequate time for the family to come to terms with the patient's death before withdrawal of life support measures is probably the most prudent course of action.

However, gradually, with more openness in Emirati society, the idea of limiting medical treatment deemed futile is getting more acceptance among families and physicians. This is the dominant approach taking effect without resistance in intensive care units in the UAE regarding futile treatment.

In general, the physicians' opinion plays a major role in managing terminally ill patients. The patient's age, diagnosis, prognosis, length of ICU stay and religious factors have been identified as factors that formulate opinions on the patient's code status (Rahman *et al.* 2012). In the Middle East, especially in the UAE, physicians have to consider religious and cultural issues more than economic considerations when making decisions for end-of-life patients. The patient in the UAE has no autonomy whatsoever; for example, if the head of a family is terminally ill, the eldest son would be the decision maker.

The development of written institutional policy is an important step towards the establishment of a formal and reasonable process for reaching an informed decision and dealing with futile treatments. Intensive care providers from varying training backgrounds and seniority levels in the Middle East agree on most of the issues on managing terminally ill patients. Limiting medical treatment in the case of medical futility is a new concept in the United Arab Emirates with no legal definition. Therefore, there may be ambiguity in interpreting the terms "no code" and "comfort care" among physicians. Euthanasia is not acceptable culturally and legally. The most acceptable form in dealing with medical futility is to limit further medical interventions. Formulating a national policy based on physicians' attitudes and the perceptions of patients and families is necessary to clarify the legal position on end-of-life decisions in general and medical futility in particular.

REFERENCES

Abuhasna S, Rahman M, Shihab Z, Bloushi A, and Chedid F. 2009. An opinion survey of family members on foregoing treatment in critically ill patients at a tertiary care center in United Arab Emirates. *Chest* 136: 39S-h-39S.

Administration of Islamic Research and Ifta. 1988. Riyadh, KSA, in Fatwa No. 12086 issued on 30.6.1409 (Hijra).

Albar M. 1996. Islamic ethics of organ transplantation and brain death. *Saudi Journal of Kidney Diseases and Transplantation* 7: 109–114.

Blair I and Sharif A. 2012. Population structure and the burden of disease in the United Arab Emirates. *Journal of Epidemiology and Global Health* 2: 61–71.

Da Costa DE, Ghazal H, and Al Khusaiby S. 2002. Do Not Resuscitate orders and ethical decisions in a neonatal intensive care unit in a Muslim community. *Archives of Disease in Childhood: Fetal and Neonatal Edition* 86: F115–119.

Damghi N, Belayachi J, Aggoug B *et al.* 2011. Withholding and withdrawing life-sustaining therapy in a Moroccan Emergency Department: An observational study. *BMC Emergency Medicine* 11, doi:10.1186/1471–227X-11–12.

Fatwa No. 115104. Cases in which it is permissible not to use resuscitation equipment (Al-Ḥālāt allatī yajūz fīhā raf' ajhiza al-in'āsh). Available at: http://www.islamqa.com/ar/ref/115104 [Accessed October 8, 2012].

Islamic Jurists 1990. Second decision on the subject of death and withdrawal of life saving equipment from the patient (Al-qarar al-thani bi-sha'n mawdu' taqrir husul al-wafat wa rafajhizat al-in'ash min jism al-insan). *Journal of Modern Fiqh Discussion* 4: 159–160.

Mobeireek A, Al-Kassimi F, Al-Zahrani K *et al.* 2008. Information disclosure and decision-making: The Middle East versus the Far East and the West. *Journal of Medical Ethics* 34: 225–229.

Rahman M, Abuhasna S, and Abuzidan F. 2012. Care of terminally-ill patients: An opinion survey among critical care healthcare providers in the Middle East. *African Health Sciences Journal* (in press).

Sachedina A. 2005. End-of-life: The Islamic view. *The Lancet* 366: 774–779.

Sprung CL, Cohen SL, Sjokvist P *et al*. 2003. End-of-life practices in European intensive care units: The Ethicus Study. *JAMA* 290: 790–797.

Takrouri MSM and Halwani TM. 2008. An Islamic medical and legal prospective of do not resuscitate order in critical care medicine. *The Internet Journal of Health* 7.

UAE National Bureau of Statistics. 2010 statistics. Available at: http://www.uaes-tatistics.gov.ae/ [Accessed October 8, 2012].

CHAPTER THIRTEEN

MEDICAL FUTILITY IN IRAN

Alireza Bagheri

SUMMARY

Medical futility is a controversial issue not only in its definition but also in its applications. The aim of medicine, if defined clearly, would determine when medical intervention for a particular case is meaningful and when it is futile.

In Islamic society, religious beliefs are a fundamental part of both personal and social life and a major determinant for healthcare decision making, especially at the end of life.

The Islamic Republic of Iran has a relatively young population, but because of the scarcity of health resources, the decision about end-of-life patients in general, and medical futility in particular, is among crucial decision making in healthcare settings. In Iran, public health services are provided through a nation-wide network with a referral system and the majority of people have insurance coverage; however, it only covers a fraction of their medical cost. There are also several active NGOs in providing support for end-of-life patients across the country. Backed by the traditional paternalistic view, physicians are in favor of unilateral decision making about medical futility and willing only to inform the patient's family about their decision. At present, however, there is a lack of regulations or guidelines to help healthcare professionals in decision making about futile treatment. In an empirical survey on medical futility in Iran, healthcare professionals have expressed four factors — scarcity of medical resources, the patient's suffering, family, and religious concerns — as very influential in their decision about futile treatment.

INTRODUCTION

End-of-life decisions, especially the decision to withdraw or withhold treatment for critically ill patients, are complex. Medical futility refers to the inappropriate application of medical intervention that is unlikely to produce any significant benefit for the patient. However, the problem of medical futility has caused controversy over not only how to define the concept of futility, but also when and how to apply it (Bagheri 2008). This controversial issue has divided experts in the relevant fields into two groups. On one side, the proponents of medical futility defend the physicians' exclusive right to determine the futility of treatment and decide whether treatment should be withheld or withdrawn (Schneiderman *et al.* 1990). On the other side, opponents argue that medical futility is a construct intended in part to give physicians more power in a context in which medical authority is threatened (Carnevale 1998). By distinction between facts and values, they believe that even the so-called factual judgment of futility has evaluative components and they argue that "physician unilateral decision making on the basis of futility is a problematic and misguided approach to the challenge of setting appropriate limits in medicine" (Rubin 1998).

In the clinical setting conflicts may arise when physicians decide to withdraw or withhold aggressive medical intervention but patients or their families request for what the physicians believe is futile treatment. In fact, in such situations, physicians and patients differ on the goals of treatment and do not agree on whether the requested treatments are beneficial.

The aim of medicine, if defined clearly, would determine when medical intervention for a particular case is meaningful and when it is futile. This would guide healthcare professionals on how vigorously to treat and when it is morally permissible to withhold or withdraw life-sustaining treatment. However, the controversy about the aim of medicine gives different answers to this question. Therefore, the controversy about medical futility, in its definition and implication, refers partly to the controversy over the aim of medicine. On the other hand, the goal of treatment is determined by the aim of medicine and this is one of the main reasons that in futility decisions, disagreement happens between families and physicians, because they do not agree on what is beneficial for the patient; "benefit from treatment" has different meanings in their views.

This chapter presents the complexity of the issue of medical futility in Iran. By providing information about the Iranian healthcare system, it explains how in an Islamic society end-of-life decisions are made and how physicians in Iran make decisions about futile treatments.

The Islamic Republic of Iran is the eighteenth-largest country in the world with 1,648,195 km^2 and stands as the seventeenth-most populous country in the world with a population of around 79 million, more than 65% of which live in urban areas.

Iran is a Muslim country and Islam has introduced its moral, ethical, and social framework for human life. It has granted a certain privilege to saving a human's life. Before Islam (625 AD), Iranians were Zoroastrian, and religious teaching emphasized the behavior and character of medical doctors. Reviewing the flourishing time of Iranian (Irani) medicine in medieval times, we see a great deal of attention paid to the ethical issues in medicine by the Iranian physicians such as Razes (865–925 AD) and Avicenna (Ibn Sina) (980–1038) in their teachings and medical practices. Persian literature, philosophy, medicine, astronomy, mathematics, and arts became major elements of Muslim civilization. After the introduction of Islam, based on Islamic teachings which govern all aspects of society, Muslim physicians put more emphasis on ethical values in their medical practice.

In Islam, the issue of life and death is among the most sensitive and is a profound ethical and judicial subject and end-of-life decision making is one of the most emotionally and ethically charged issues in Islamic society. Based on the importance of Islamic opinions on different bioethical issues, Islamic scholars are involved in the discussion of ethical issues in medicine such as end-of-life decisions, abortion, artificial reproductive technologies, brain death and organ transplantation. There are some Islamic principles that are instrumental to healthcare decision making, for instance principles such as "do no harm" (*la dharar wa la dherar*), the principle of "necessity" (*dharura*), and the principle of "no hardship" have been referenced in policy making regarding end-of-life issues. The Iranian Charter of Patient Rights which has been recently adopted by the Ministry of Health and Medical Education has addressed some of the critical issues in providing healthcare at the end of life (Parsapour *et al.* 2010).

It should be noted that Iran has a relatively young population, but because of the scarcity of health resources, the issues of end of life and decision making regarding futile care are among important topics in healthcare settings. Although healthcare professionals have stressed the importance and usefulness of regulations or guidelines, there is no regulation or guideline to deal with futile treatments.

THE HEALTHCARE SYSTEM IN IRAN

The Constitution of the Islamic Republic of Iran, in Articles 29 and 43, emphasizes the highest level of health as a fundamental right for its citizens. The Ministry of Health and Medical Education is in charge of fulfilling this goal through the implementation of the national health policies. The Ministry delegates the implementation of the policies through the public medical universities across the country. There is at least one medical university in every province. The Chancellor of each medical university is the highest health authority and the minister's deputy in the province, who is responsible for the public health, healthcare provision, and medical education. In Iran, healthcare and public health services are provided through a nation-wide network. This network consists of a referral system, starting at health houses in rural areas, primary healthcare centers, health posts in urban regions, and going through secondary-level hospitals in the cities and provincial capitals and tertiary hospitals operating in large cities.

The public sector provides primary, secondary, and tertiary health services; however, the focus of the government on primary healthcare over the last two decades has made the government the main provider of primary healthcare services. Some primary healthcare services such as prenatal care and vaccination are free of charge in public facilities.

In rural areas, health services are provided free of charge based on medical protocols and standardized packages. However, still this coverage is not complete and almost 10% of the rural population has no access to this service. In urban areas, especially big cities, there are more than one medical university responsible to provide services, which causes confusion over the administrative districts (Shadpour 2006).

The public sector also provides a considerable part of secondary and tertiary health services and plays a significant role in the healthcare system in Iran, but it mainly focuses on secondary and tertiary healthcare in urban areas. There are also many active nongovernmental organizations (NGOs) in healthcare; however, these NGOs are mainly active in special diseases such as children's cancer, breast cancer, diabetes, and thalassemia.

Iran has increased investment in healthcare during the last 10 years, and total expenditure on health as a percentage of gross domestic production (GDP) has increased from 4.7% in 1995 to 7.8% in 2006 (Mehrdad 2009). Accordingly, almost all health investment indices have improved since the last decade. It should be noted that the Iranian Development Plan set the goal for out-of-pocket payment to as low as 30% in 2008. Nonetheless, almost 55% of health spending, in spite of government spending on health, is still paid out of pocket by patients. The outpatient treatment proportion of health funds is 18%, inpatient treatment 33%, and the primary care proportion is only 7% (Sabbagh 2004).

According to the health insurance system's official data, more than 90% of Iranian people are under the coverage of at least one kind of health insurance, public or private insurance. However, one survey shows that 26% of Iranians do not have any kind of medical insurance (Naghavi 2004). There are four types of public health insurance in the country. The first is the Social Security Organization, which is one of the largest health insurers in Iran. It covers people who are nongovernment employees. More than 27 million workers and their families are under this insurance coverage. Almost 30% of the workers' income goes to this organization to provide resources for this insurance system. This organization owns and runs many clinics and hospitals in the country. Medical services in these clinics and hospitals are offered either free of charge or at very low cost for insured people.

The second is the Medical Services Insurance Organization, which provides health insurance to government employees, students, and rural dwellers. This system covers 6.7 million governmental employees and their family, who pay a fixed amount each month for their insurance. The government pays the villagers' total premium and 80% of the students' premium. Most of the healthcare providers accept this kind of medical insurance but patients should pay a part of the medical cost.

The third includes organizations such as the Oil Ministry, banks, municipalities, and military organizations that provide health insurance for their own employees.

The Imam Khomeini Relief Foundation (Committee) is the fourth, which provides health insurance for the uninsured poor people, and the government contributes to their premium through this organization's fund.

There are also some semi-public insurance companies, which mainly cover co-payments for costly inpatient services. It should be noted that for cancer patients there are some governmental subsidies, as well as support for end-of-life patients by NGOs and charity organizations; however, there is no data to show the end-of-life expenditure in Iran and the efficiency of these subsidies. A small percentage of Iranian people are not covered by any of these health insurance plans. It should be noted that different insurance systems provide different levels of service coverage and some people have enrolled in two different health insurance plans to make it easier to shop for services at lower cost. However, with all these insurance plans, there are individuals with no insurance coverage. Several NGOs and charity organizations also provide help to end-of-life patients and their families. For instance, the Charity Foundation for Special Diseases was set up in 1997 as a nongovernmental organization to support patients suffering from special diseases such as cancer, multiple sclerosis, thalassemia, and many other life-threatening health problems. Since then almost 54,000 patients have received support through three medical centers in Tehran and many others across the country under the foundation. There are also other NGOs in Iran which support end-stage patients and their families such as The Society for Helping the Cancer Patients and the Society to Support Children Suffering from Cancer (MAHAK), which is particularly responsible for the reduction of the child mortality rate and the burden of cancer on children and their families. During the past two decades, this organization has built a highly specialized hospital and research center in pediatrics to help those children at the end of their lives.

END-OF-LIFE ISSUES IN IRAN

The rapid advances in biomedical technology and its applications have raised ethical questions, especially at the end of life. Dying patients face complex and unique challenges that threaten their physical, psychological, and spiritual integrity. Decisions about withholding and withdrawing life-sustaining treatment, the patient's quality of life, futile treatment, and allocation of scarce health resources are among these issues. However, the educational background of healthcare providers is frequently not strong enough to respond to these issues appropriately. The social understanding of the concepts of health, disease, life, and death influences the society's reflection on end-of-life issues. It also shapes related legislation and guidelines. Many authors have stated that the definition of human death is beyond the scope of medicine alone, and philosophical, cultural, and religious issues have a great role (Bagheri 2007). Therefore, formulation of a proper definition of death requires an understanding of the religious estimation of human life and an endeavor to unravel the secrets of the soul or the spirit, which, according to Muslim belief, departs the body at the time of death (Sachedina 2009). In Iranian society, religious beliefs are a fundamental part of personal as well as social life and a major factor in healthcare decision making, especially at the end of life. Therefore, it is appropriate to provide some information about Islamic views on human life and death.

The Qur'anic Views on the Beginning and End of Human Life

Regarding the creation and nature of the human being, God the Glorified says in the Holy Qur'an:

> "And certainly We created man of an extract of clay. Then We made him a small seed in a firm resting-place. Then We made the seed a clot, then We made the clot a lump of bones. Then We clothed the bones with flesh, then We caused it to grow into another creation, so blessed be Allah, the best of the creators" (23:12–14).

Thus, God says that the human being is at his initial creation nothing except a material body that has undergone various forms from its earliest existence, until God the Almighty causes the very corporeal and material being to grow into another "creation" in which the human being acquires perception and will so much so that he is enabled to do things, such as thinking, that could not be done by a mere body.

God also says: "So when I have made him complete and breathed into him of My spirit, fall down making obeisance to him" (15:29).

Thus, the Almighty God has composed the human being of two components: matter and pure essence or the very soul or spirit that is spiritual and immaterial. These two components will remain together as long as the human being continues to live in this world. As soon as he dies, his body will die but his soul will survive. The human being, whose truth is his very soul, will return to God the Glorified. As God says: "Then after that you will most surely die. Then surely on the day of resurrection you shall be raised" (23:15–16).

In other words, the body and soul are truly companions. Like dough that is made of flour and water, the human being is also made of these two components: body and soul. When the soul accompanies the body, that person embraces life, and when they separate from each other, such separation means death (Tabatabaee 1984).

The Concept of Death in the Holy Qur'an

As mentioned, the concept of death and its definition influences people's understanding and decisions related to the end of life. This concept in a religious society such as Iran is based on Islamic teachings. In the Islamic view, the issue of death and life is one of the reasons for monotheism. Neither can life and death be removed from the world nor can they be said to have occurred on their own. Hence, death and life need an efficient cause, and God the Almighty is their efficient cause. The Holy Qur'an considers death an evolutionary process in the existence, not non-existence and annihilation. The human being passes from the world of nature to the other World, and this, getting rid of the world, is called death. Thus this transfer from this world to the Hereafter is called death, but death does not bring about annihilation (Javadi Amoli 1987).

The Holy Qur'an regards death as God's creation. Hence, it reads: "(He) created death and life that He may try you — which of you is best in deeds" (117:6).

Death and life are both at God's control. As the Qur'an reads: "And He it is Who causes death and gives life" (103:44). If death were at the hands of others, they could prevent it, as human beings have always been thinking how to prevent death and trying to avoid dying. However, the Qur'an reads: "Every soul must taste of death" (21:35).

It should be noted that the current notion of the right to die, which has been accepted in some societies, is not recognized in Islam. Based on the Islamic Shari'a the decision regarding the end of life is through divine decree and it refuses to recognize individual rights in this matter (Sachedina 2005). According to the Qur'an, life is a divine trust and cannot be terminated by any form of human intervention. Its term has been fixed by the unalterable divine decree. The Holy Qur'an reads: "God takes the souls at the time of their death" (39:42). Therefore, the right to be assisted in dying is also ruled out.

The juridical principle of non-maleficence that states "no harm shall be inflicted or reciprocated in Islam (*la darar wa la dirar fi'l-islam*)" provides the justification of this ruling.

When death approaches, the close family and friends try to support and comfort the dying person through supplication as well as remembrance of Allah and His will. The attendance is to help the dying person to repeat his commitment to the unity of God.

The recently developed Iranian Charter of Patient Rights has emphasized the special needs of a dying patient and urged healthcare providers to be sensitive to these issues. In medical practice in Iran, family authority is often more influential than the patient's autonomy. Many physicians provide information about the patient's illness, diagnosis, and prognosis to the family members first, but not to the terminally ill patient. If the family asks physicians not to tell the patient, many physicians will agree to this request, and many patients accept this as standard practice. Therefore, it can be claimed that decision making in healthcare is a family-centered model. However, based on cultural changes as well as the Patient Rights Charter which emphasizes patient autonomy, this practice has been challenged, and there are many patients who would ask for more disclosure from their physicians.

In the case of end-of-life decision making when a person lacks the capacity for making a decision in Islamic societies, the family has been given the right to decide on behalf of their beloved ones based on his/her best interest especially if the patient did not express his wishes. In the case of minors, also parents can act as a surrogate decision maker for their children. In the case of emergencies and unconsciousness, accompanying family members act as surrogates.

DEALING WITH MEDICAL FUTILITY IN CLINICAL SETTINGS

In Iran, compared to the United States, which has a history of almost three decades of discussion on medical futility, the issue is relatively in its primary stage. However, although as mentioned earlier Iran has a relatively young population, the problem of scarce health resources has given decision making about medical futility a very critical bioethical priority.

In the healthcare system, there is a lack of regulation or any guidelines to help physicians in dealing with such a sensitive issue. However, dealing with this dilemma is a common situation in end-of-life care and both duties — to treat and care and not to prolong death — should be considered carefully. It is noteworthy that the primary obligation of a Muslim doctor is to provide care and reduce pain. Therefore, the challenge associated with the decision about futile treatment and the use of palliative care at the end of life remains. For example, healthcare providers sometimes struggle with how to use pain medication appropriately for terminally ill patients because treating the patient's pain sufficiently may potentially hasten the patient's death. As the decision making in healthcare settings is a family-centered model in Iran, in general, withholding and withdrawing life support should be discussed with the family and if the treating physician finds a certain modality of treatment useless or increasing the suffering of the patient, that modality of treatment should not be enforced from the beginning. An essential principle in Islam is that human life has infinite value, and issues such as aging, health, illness, and death are considered natural parts of human life and individuals are responsible for their bodies, which belong to God. The end of life for a dying patient should be as smooth as possible and any unnecessary invasive procedures that could bring suffering to the dying patient or his relatives should never be used. Withholding and withdrawing life support interventions deemed futile is a controversial issue in Iran. In dealing with a terminally ill patient, different juridical schools of Islam ruled that when an invasive treatment is necessary to save the patient's life, life-saving equipment cannot be turned off unless the physicians are certain about the inevitability of death. On the other hand, Islam recognizes that death is an inevitable part of human existence so unnecessary treatment should not be provided if it prolongs the final stages (death) of a terminal illness. It recognizes the possibility of arriving at a collective decision by those involved in providing care, including the attending physician and the family, to withhold or withdraw life support intervention deemed futile. Therefore, a great challenge is to define the moment when there is no hope for life and the dying process has begun. In recognition of the fact that not all medical interventions at the end of life are necessary, the healthcare system has recently been emphasizing the importance of palliative and hospice care for terminally ill patients. Although the main reason might be better allocation of limited resources, this in some way is an appropriate way to avoid medical intervention deemed futile.

Three years ago, the first hospice was established in a large cancer institute at Tehran University of Medical Sciences to offer palliative care to terminal patients for whom medical interventions are futile. To address the needs of those patients, palliative care and hospices are expanding across the country.

MEDICAL FUTILITY: WHO DECIDES?

For many Muslims, religious beliefs are a fundamental part of both personal and social existence in their daily life and a major determinant for healthcare decision making, especially at the end of life. In Islamic teachings, the importance of inter-human as well as human-divine relations has been emphasized and Muslims look at these teachings to shape their relationship with others and the Almighty God. This understanding is the basis for their end-of-life decision making. As was noted earlier, family authority is often more influential than the patient's autonomy.

In addition, based on the dominancy of medical paternalism in healthcare settings, the general concept is that all decisions at the end of life are in the domain of medical expertise. This general idea among physicians supports medical futility only based on the concept of physiological futility and tries to ignore medical futility as a value judgment (qualitative futility). Therefore, physicians tend to believe that they have a unilateral decision-making authority not only in any matters regarding the patient's care, but also regarding end-of-life care and medical futility.

An empirical study confirms this willingness for unilateral decision making. In this study, regarding who can make the decision, the majority responded that it is the responsibility of the physician in charge to make a futility decision. However, they emphasized the importance of consultation with a colleague about medical futility (Bagheri 2011). This study shows that in case of disagreement between physician and patient/family, the hospital ethics committee can be used as a resource to resolve the disagreement about futile treatment.

If the patient lacks the capacity for decision making, which is quite frequent in clinical practice with end-of-life patients, in Islamic societies the family has the right to decide on behalf of their loved ones, based on his/her best interest, especially if the patient did not express his/her wishes. In the case of minors, parents are surrogate decision makers for their children. In such cases, physicians would communicate with the family members to inform them of their futility decision.

As mentioned, the notion of the right to die has not been recognized, and therefore patients' informed decisions and voluntary requests for ending their lives have no legitimacy and physician-assisted death has no place in clinical decision making.

Physicians' Attitudes Towards Medical Futility in Iran

In order to collect some empirical data about medical futility in Iran, the author conducted a study in 2011. The aim was to document medical professionals' opinions about medical futility; its definition as well as its application in healthcare settings in Iran. In this study, first, to document physicians' opinions about medical futility a semi-structured interview among 12 medical specialists from different fields in medicine was conducted.

Regarding the definition of medical futility, there was controversy not only regarding how to define it but also what would be a correct translation of medical futility in the Persian language. There was a consensus among interviewees that in evaluating futile treatment, the approach should be case by case and there was no possibility to develop a general diagnostic protocol for all patients in futility decisions. Regarding who could make the decision, the majority believed that it was the responsibility of the physician in charge to make a decision about whether the treatment at hand was futile or not. However, the importance of consultation with a colleague when making decisions on medical futility was emphasized. Among them, one of the participants expressed that in Iran, the hospital was also responsible for hospitalized patients, and therefore the physician in charge should report the case to the medical director of the hospital. They also emphasized the role of the family in decision making. A question was asked about hospitals' interest in continuing futile treatment in order to make more money, especially in private hospitals; in response, the participants did not deny the possibility of such incentives to over-treat. However, they believed that managing such an end-of-life case would be so complicated and burdensome for physicians that they would never decide to keep the patient in the hospital and continue providing futile treatment for that incentive.

When asked about the influential factors in futility decisions, the interviewees listed four main factors: scarcity of medical resources, the patient's suffering, accommodating the family, and religious concerns.

A question was raised to see if the experts believed that developing a policy or guideline would be useful for physicians in dealing with medical futility. In response, they all said they believed that it would be helpful for decision making and would help physicians to defend their futility decision when talking to the patients' family. However, one of them raised concerns about the legality of such a policy and whether the policy or guidelines would be supported by legislation. One of the interviewees also was concerned about the working group or committee members who would be responsible for making the policy or guidelines. Two interviewees emphasized that such guidelines would be very instrumental in futility decisions if allocation of scarce resources were at stake.

About the involvement of hospital ethics committees in futility decisions, their opinions were divers. For example, some were concerned that in Iran, hospital ethics committees were not well developed and therefore the concern was whether those committees had the capacity and expertise to be helpful in this regard. They had different opinions on whether physicians must request for the ethics committee's involvement in consultation and decision making or whether they should only notify the ethics committee about the case and decision made. Another issue raised was about the appropriate time at which the hospital ethics committee should be notified, i.e. as soon as the case happens or afterward. When asked whether in medicine there was a point beyond which it could be claimed that continuing treatment was just delaying the process of the patient's death and not prolonging the patient's life, they said they believed that in medical practice, a distinction should be made between an intervention that may prolong life, from interventions that only delay death and cause suffering. However, they also referred to the religious perspective and said that this should be checked with religious experts as well. One of the participants, who had an extensive religious background, said that delaying the patient's death in itself was prolonging life and had to be followed.

In the next step of the study, two group discussions were organized to discuss the issue in more detail. Participants were mostly medical specialists as well as experts in law, ethics, and Islamic Shari'a. A question was designed to discuss physicians' authority for unilateral decision making on futile medicine. The consensus was that physicians should have such an authority for decision making. However, they emphasized that because of the sensitivity of the issue as well as the importance of the patient's/ family's trust, it was better to consult with another physician for a second opinion. Regarding the hospital ethics committee's involvement, they said that first the physician should communicate with the patient's family, and in case of disagreement between them, the issue could be referred to the hospital ethics committee to resolve the disagreement. In this part of the study, a model on how to approach medical futility in clinical settings was developed. In both group discussions, participants emphasized the importance of education for medical professionals on medical futility and decision making.

The last part of the study was a consultative workshop which discussed and finalized the suggested model for cases of medical futility. According to the suggested model, the physician should inform the patient/family about his futility decision and, if they accept the physician's decision, they can proceed based on their shared decision. In case of disagreement between physician and patient/family, the case can be referred to the hospital ethics committee. To resolve the problem, in the first step, the committee can hold a meeting with the patient's family and other involved parties. Accordingly, if the patient/family accepts the physician's decision, it will be considered a shared decision, and if not, the hospital ethics committee will provide its recommendation to the parties involved. The consensus was that the ethics committee's recommendation would be followed.

RELATED LAW AND REGULATIONS

In Iran, the interaction between health policy makers and religious leaders has established a framework to develop related legislation in healthcare, such as reproductive health, abortion, brain death and organ transplantation, as well as end-of-life decision making.

Currently, there is no particular law or regulation to govern medical futility in Iran as there is a lack of professional guidelines on how to deal with futile treatments. However, the necessity of having a medical protocol or guidelines to help them in futility decision making is getting more attention among physicians as well as healthcare policy makers.

In terms of end-of-life issues in general, the Iranian Patient Rights Charter can be cited as a new set of developed guidelines helping patients, their family, and healthcare professionals to deal with the end of life properly. The Patient Rights Charter was compiled with a comprehensive approach in 2009 and adopted by the Ministry of Health and Medical Education. This Charter aims to elucidate the rights of recipients of health services as well as observing ethical standards in medicine. The Charter has been formulated in the framework of 5 chapters and 37 articles including its vision and an explanatory note. The Charter's five chapters are on (1) the right of receiving suitable services, (2) the right to access to desirable and enough information, (3) the right to choose and to decide freely about receiving healthcare, (4) the right to privacy and confidentiality, and finally (5) the right to access an efficient system of dealing with complaints which are explained in Articles 14, 9, 7, 4, and 3, respectively (Parsapour *et al.* 2010). Chapter 1 of the Charter emphasizes that "Every individual has the right to receive appropriate health care services" with "respecting human dignity, cultural values, and religious beliefs". In dealing with terminally ill patients at the end of life, it calls for "providing comfort for terminally ill patients if death is imminent. Comfort refers to decreasing patients' suffering and pain, to observe their mental, social, spiritual and moral requirements at the time of death. Dying patients are entitled to be accompanied by a person of their choice."

As mentioned earlier, the definition of death affects some health policies, especially end-of-life policies such as futile treatment and withdrawal of life-sustaining treatment. In terms of brain death, in Iran, the notion of brain death as an alternative to human death has not been recognized in the legislation called the Brain Death and Organ Transplantation Act. The Act, which was ratified by the Parliament in 2000, authorizes organ removal for transplantation from a brain-dead patient without confirming that brain death is equal to human death. Therefore, the ventilator can be withdrawn from a brain-dead patient, not because he is a dead person, or providing treatment is futile, but because his organs can be transplanted to another patient with his prior consent. However, if the case is not a suitable candidate for organ donation, this Act cannot be applied and it falls into a gray zone and is subject to controversy in decision making.

END-OF-LIFE CARE AND EUTHANASIA

In Islamic society, the concept of the right to die as it has been acknowledged in Western society has not been accepted. According to the Qur'an, life is a divine trust and cannot be terminated by any form of human intervention. Its term has been fixed by the unalterable divine decree. The Holy Qur'an reads: "God takes the souls at the time of their death" (39:42). Since the end-of-life decision is through divine decree, the Islamic Shari'a refuses to recognize the individual's right in that matter (Sachedina 2005). Therefore the current notion of the right to die has not been recognized; and the right to be assisted in dying, whether through passive or active means, is also ruled out. The juridical principle of non-maleficence that states "no harm shall be inflicted or reciprocated in Islam" (*la darar wa la dirar fi'l-islam*) provides the justification of this ruling. Therefore, it is impossible to justify the euthanasia decision from a religious point of view. From a strict theological viewpoint, suicide trades a transient, unbearable life in this world for an even more horrible, eternal one beyond. In the Shari'a such actions are forbidden, along with less drastic measures of self-harm (Sachedina 2009, p. 169).

There are, however, two situations in the treatment that could be interpreted as passive assistance in allowing a terminally ill patient to die, as Sachedina explains. The first is using painkillers to relieve physical pain and psychological distress, with no intention to kill the patient, but which could shorten the patient's life. As long as the situation does not involve an intention to cause death, a medical intervention to provide necessary treatment for the relief of pain or other symptoms of serious physical distress is not regarded as criminal and is permitted in Islamic law. The second situation is in relation to withdrawing treatment, whether pursuant to a refusal of a death-delaying treatment or through mutual and informed decision making by patient, physician, and other parties involved in providing care for the patient. Although in this case there is an intention to allow the person to die when it is certain that death will result from its omission, this is not a culpable act under Islamic law. According to him, there are no other grounds for the justifiable ending of a terminally ill person's life, whether through voluntary active euthanasia or physician-assisted suicide (Sachedina 2009, p. 170).

About suicide, the Qur'an is very clear: "do not kill yourselves as God has been to you very merciful" (4:29). Taking away life should be the domain of the One who gives life. There is pain and suffering at the terminal end of an illness, but there is reward from God for those who patiently persevere in suffering (39:10 and 31). Therefore, there is no room for suicide or assisted suicide in Islam.

A study among patients in Tehran university hospitals in 2009 showed that these patients had some degree of acceptance about passive voluntary euthanasia (Hasanzade-Hadad et al. 2011).

Another study, which was a descriptive-analytical study among 233 students at Tehran University, showed that the acceptance of euthanasia was very low (Aghababaei et al. 2011). A study among 20 specialist medical doctors who work with end-of-life patients showed that there is a diversity in the definition of an end-of-life patient among different specialists; for example a neurologist defines it as a brain-dead patient while a nephrologist considers a chronic renal patient as an end-of-life patient. But almost all participants emphasized the role of the patient's family and the physician's clinical judgment in decision making (Kazemian 2008).

In the Islamic tradition, instead of contemplating ways to end one's life, either by refusal of life-support treatment or by requesting to die with active assistance, Muslims afflicted with illness are advised to ask God to forgive their sins and pray for an opportunity to have a fresh start with restored health. In the current discussion about passive euthanasia and medical futility, the main question is at what point medical intervention can be considered a delay in the process of the patient's death, instead of prolonging the patient's life. However, in Iran, a challenge for physicians in dealing with medical futility is how to convince the patient's family that withholding futile care is not euthanasia. The intention is not to hasten death; it is, instead, to accept death, in a reasonable and peaceful manner.

CONCLUSION

In the Islamic Republic of Iran, the issue of medical futility in clinical settings is gaining more attention, not because of the aging population but because of the scarcity of health resources.

This article showed how, in an Islamic society such as Iran, religious beliefs are fundamental in end-of-life decision making. The understanding of the concepts of health, disease, life, and death shape our understanding of the aim of medicine and determine how far medical interventions are necessary and useful and when they are futile. Based on the traditional paternalistic view, with the predominant model of the physician-patient relationship, there is a tendency among physicians toward unilateral decision making about medical futility. Nonetheless, consulting with a colleague about futility decisions and informing the patient's family about the decision have been considered important in dealing with these cases.

In making decisions about futile treatment the four primary factors influencing decisions are the scarcity of medical resources, the patient's suffering, accommodating the family, and most importantly religious concerns about impermissibly hastening death. In dealing with medical futility, it is crucial to develop professional guidelines. In addition to guidelines, however, there is a great need for professional as well as public education about end-of-life issues in general and medical futility in particular.

REFERENCES

Aghababaei N, Hatami J, and Rostami R. 2011. The role of individual characteristics and judgment pattern in attitude toward euthanasia. *Iranian Journal of
Critical Care Nursing* 4: 23–32 (in Persian).

Bagheri A. 2007. Individual choice in the definition of death. *Journal of Medical
Ethics* 33: 146–149.

Bagheri A. 2008. Regulating medical futility: Neither physician's paternalism, nor
excessive patient's autonomy. *European Journal of Health Law* 15: 45–53.

Bagheri A. 2011. Medical futility decision making guidelines. Research Report,
Proposal No. 89–01–50–10201, submitted to Tehran University of Medical
Sciences (in Persian).

Carnevale FA. 1998. The utility of futility: The construction of bioethical problems. *Nursing Ethics* 5: 509–517.

Hasanzade-Hadad A, Rastegary H, Sedaghat M *et al.* 2011. Evaluation of Tehran
University patients' attitude toward euthanasia. *Iranian Journal of Medical
Ethics and History of Medicine* 4: 33–41 (in Persian).

Holy Qur'an. All references to the Holy Qur'an have been quoted from Shakir
MH, trans. 1990. *Holy Qur'an.* Qum: Anssarian Publications.

Javadi Amoli A. 1987. *Tafseer-e mozu'ee-ye Qur'an-e Kareem* (Topical interpretation of the Holy Qur'an), Vol. 2. Raja Publications, p. 397 (in Persian).

Kazemian A. 2008. Physician's attitude about terminal patients. *Iranian Journal
of Medical Ethics and History of Medicine* 2: 61–68.

Mehrdad R. 2009. Health system in Iran. *Japan Medical Association Journal*
52: 69–73.

Naghavi M and Jamshidi HR. 2004. *Utilization of Health Service in Islamic
Republic of Iran.* Tehran: Ministry of Health and Medical Education.

Organ Transplantation Act. 2000. Parliament of the IR Iran, Deceased or Brain
Dead Patients Organ Transplantation Act (No. H/24804-T/9929). The execu-
tive bylaw of this Act was proposed by the Ministry of Health and Medical
Education and approved by the Cabinet Council on May 15, 2002. (IR Iran
Cabinet Council: Executive Bylaw of Deceased or Brain Dead Patients OT.
H/24804-T/9929. May 15, 2002).

Parsapour A, Bagheri A, and Larijani B. 2010. Patient Rights Charter in Iran.
Journal of Medical Ethics and History of Medicine Special Issue 3: 39–47
(in Persian).

Rubin SB. 1998. *When Doctors Say No: The Battleground of Medical Futility.* Bloomington, IN: Indiana University Press, pp. 88–91.

Sabbagh Kermani M. 2004. Health care financing in Iran. Final Report. APW No. 03/144. MOH & ME/WHO, February, p. 37.

Sachedina A. 2005. End-of-life: The Islamic view. *The Lancet* 366: 774–779.

Sachedina A. 2009. *Islamic Biomedical Ethics.* Oxford: Oxford University Press, pp. 146, 169–170.

Schneiderman LJ, Jecker NS, and Jonsen AR. 1990. Medical futility: Its meaning and ethical implications. *Annals of Internal Medicine* 112: 949–954.

Shadpour K. 2006. Health sector reform in the Islamic Republic of Iran. *Hakim Research Journal* 9: 1–18 (in Persian).

Tabatabaee SM. 1984. *Al-mizan*, Vol. 20. Islami Publications, p. 222 (in Arabic).

INDEX